The Carmichael Training Systems Cyclist's Diary

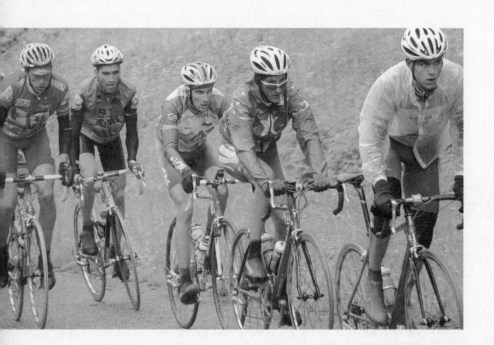

The Carmichael Training Systems Cyclist's Diary

Chris Carmichael
with Jim Rutberg

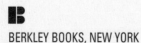

BERKLEY BOOKS, NEW YORK

THE BERKLEY PUBLISHING GROUP
Published by the Penguin Group
Penguin Group (USA) Inc.
375 Hudson Street, New York, New York 10014, USA
Penguin Group (Canada), 10 Alcorn Avenue, Toronto, Ontario M4V 3B2, Canada
(a division of Pearson Penguin Canada Inc.)
Penguin Books Ltd., 80 Strand, London WC2R 0RL, England
Penguin Group Ireland, 25 St. Stephen's Green, Dublin 2, Ireland (a division of Penguin Books Ltd.)
Penguin Group (Australia), 250 Camberwell Road, Camberwell, Victoria 3124, Australia
(a division of Pearson Australia Group Pty. Ltd.)
Penguin Books India Pvt. Ltd., 11 Community Centre, Panchsheel Park, New Delhi—110 017, India
Penguin Group (NZ), Cnr. Airborne and Rosedale Roads, Albany, Auckland 1310, New Zealand
(a division of Pearson New Zealand Ltd.)
Penguin Books (South Africa) (Pty.) Ltd., 24 Sturdee Avenue, Rosebank, Johannesburg 2196,
South Africa

Penguin Books Ltd., Registered Offices: 80 Strand, London WC2R 0RL, England

THE CARMICHAEL TRAINING SYSTEMS CYCLIST'S DIARY

CTS, CTS Pyramid of Success, FoundationMiles, EnduranceMiles, RecoveryMiles, Tempo,
SteadyState and ClimbingRepeats are trademarks of Carmichael Training Systems, Inc.

Copyright © 2005 Carmichael Training Systems, Inc.
Cover design by George Long
Cover photo of Lance Armstrong by Graham Watson
Cover photo of Chris Carmichael by Sigrid Estrada
Photo on title page courtesy of CTS
Book design by Tiffany Estreicher

PRINTING HISTORY
Berkley trade paperback edition / April 2005
Berkley trade paperback ISBN: 0-425-20038-8

This book has been catalogued with the Library of Congress.

PRINTED IN THE UNITED STATES OF AMERICA

10   9   8   7   6   5   4   3   2   1

Contents

Part 1:

The CTS Formula for Success

Why Keep a Training Diary?

The most successful athletes put the past to work in shaping their futures. Your training diary is a unique record of the things that worked, and the things that didn't work, in training and competition. We are all striving to achieve our goals and progress as athletes with each passing year. You are most likely stronger, faster, and more skilled than you were when you first rode a bicycle, but like every athlete, you still have room to improve. This training diary can reveal the path you took to get where you are today, and help you create an action plan for the future.

In order for your training diary to help you, it is important to consider the information you are recording. While the number of miles or hours you ride is important, there's more to training than just accumulating time on your bike. Even adding detailed data about your training intervals doesn't make your diary complete. Data itself is just a mess of numbers. In order to give them meaning, you have to add subjective feelings, perceptions, and insights. Over time, this subjective information provides context for the trends you see with your training data. You can see how your relationships or stresses at work affect your training performances, how your training load affects the quality of your sleep, and how your regeneration weeks work to propel your fitness.

Training diaries serve important purposes for both short- and long-term success. Recording baseline, training, and personal data on a daily basis can help you recognize the signs of overreaching and monitor them so they don't progress into overtraining. Over the long-term, you can use the information in your training diary to compare your current fitness to where you were last year or even the year before.

On top of wanting to improve from one year to the next, you may have specific goals for a competitive event or for a short period when you want to be at your best. You can design your training program to deliver you to your goal event as a 100% Ready Athlete. The CTS Pyramid of Success™ (shown below) is the model I developed to help Lance Armstrong get back in top form after cancer and is the model CTS coaches and I use to guide athletes to the best performances of their athletic careers. Building your pyramid begins with setting goals and managing your time, and progresses through physical training, mental preparation, nutrition, skill development, and the peaking process. (The entire program is detailed in my book *The Ultimate Ride*.) This training diary is an important component of your overall plan for success, as it allows you to track your progress, adjust for challenges, and achieve the confidence that comes from knowing you're on the path to reaching your goals.

100% Ready

Peaking Process

Specialization • Confidence

Nutritional Plan • Pre, Post, During

Preparation Training • Skill Development

Aerobic Strength • Foundation and Resistance Training

Energy Systems • Components and Principles of Training • Periodization

Goal Setting • Psychological Fitness • Imagery • Stress Management • Mental Drills

THE CTS PYRAMID OF SUCCESS™

Goal Setting

Ambition is part of an athlete's nature. For some, it manifests itself as a desire to compete and win. Others desire to complete a century, lose some weight, or get to the top of a local hill more quickly. In working to reach your individual goals, you are trying to attain the feeling of accomplishment and satisfaction that comes with achieving something valuable. Your goals need to be worthwhile to you—worth the commitment and hard work you're going to devote to their accomplishment.

Before pursuing a goal you find valuable, you have to know exactly where you are in relation to it. Be honest with yourself with regard to the time you have to spend training and your current state of fitness. Both of these pieces of information will help you design the best route to your destination.

Achieving your goals requires a commitment to excellence. You need to possess the desire, determination, and self-motivation to pursue a goal you feel passionate about. Your commitment to excellence results in a more focused journey toward that goal and increases your chances of achieving it.

Take some time to think about your dreams and aspirations—this is the first step in preparing for your successful journey. Your goals will provide direction for your training. They should be specific and focused on measurable markers (power, skills), because progress toward general goals—for instance, "to ride better"—is more difficult to see. Be careful of setting goals that are tied to the results of a specific race because there are too many variables involved in competition. Instead, base your goals on things you can control, like increasing your sustainable power. Most important, you need to create and own your goals. When I say you need to "own" your goals, I mean you must think of things that you want to achieve—you and you alone. Ownership will motivate you through the tough times and make achieving your goals more rewarding.

Success begins with a dream and becomes a reality through the pursuit of well thought-out goals. Specifically, you should have short- and long-term goals; goals for today, tomorrow, next week as well as for the future—a long-term goal that everything is working toward. Set **dream goals** (ultimate and inspiring), **confidence-building goals** (midterm, ambitious but realistic), and **action goals** (here and now, details of daily workouts). And remember, these are *your* desires, ambitions, and dreams; only you can create them and only you can achieve them!

Use the goal-setting worksheets on pages 6 and 7 to help create and define your long-term and short-term goals.

Periodization

A structured and organized training program is the most effective means of reaching your goals. Systematically arranging workout and recovery days into weeks and months of goal-oriented, progressive training increases the

Basic Goal-Setting Worksheet

sample

Season/Long-term Goal:

Ride a sub–40-minute 30km time trial at Nationals

Sustained concentration and effort

GOAL EVALUATION DATE: *May 2006*

What will it take to achieve my goal?

• *A solid training plan, better start technique, solid turn-around technique*

• *Improved concentration ability*

Short-term goals that will help you achieve your long-term goal:

• *Research and hire a coach—start of November 2005.*

• *Have a solid training plan designed—end of November 2005.*

• *Use concentration exercises in sustained effort practices—evaluate after each practice.*

• *Find out as much as possible about Nationals' course—by February 2006.*

Is the long-term goal:	Are the short-term goals:
X Specific?	X Specific?
X Challenging, but realistic?	X Challenging, but realistic?
X Observable?	X Observable?
X Within your control?	X Within your control?
X Something you're committed to?	X Things you're committed to?

Basic Goal-Setting Worksheet

Season/Long-term Goal:

_____

_____

_____

GOAL EVALUATION DATE: _____

What will it take to achieve my goal?

_____

_____

_____

Short-term goals that will help you achieve your long-term goal:

_____

_____

_____

_____

Is the long-term goal:	Are the short-term goals:
__ Specific?	__ Specific?
__ Challenging, but realistic?	__ Challenging, but realistic?
__ Observable?	__ Observable?
__ Within your control?	__ Within your control?
__ Something you're committed to?	__ Things you're committed to?

likelihood that you'll reach or even exceed your expectations. The concept of **periodization** breaks the year into smaller segments, each focused on achieving a specific goal. Your training progresses from the general aspects of aerobic preparedness to specific technique and energy system work as you approach your goal event.

I break the year into four main periods: **Foundation**, **Preparation**, **Specialization**, and **Transition**. Starting with the Foundation Period, each segment of the training year builds on the accomplishments of the previous period. This means your performance in the Specialization Period is dependant upon the groundwork you laid months earlier during the Foundation Period.

The **Foundation Period** is a time of general aerobic and strength development. During this block, your training is focused on building your aerobic engine, which supports all of your other energy systems. Foundation training is characterized by a high volume of training at low to moderate intensity.

The **Preparation Period** focuses on further aerobic development as well as improving your power at lactate threshold. The volume and intensity of your training increases, and your focus narrows as you enter your competitive season. Your training during this period progresses from general conditioning to workouts designed to meet the specific demands of your competition. For many cyclists, this is the portion of the year when you notice the most significant increases in your sustainable power output.

The **Specialization Period** is the fun part of the year: it's when you're at your fastest and most powerful. Your training should address the demands of your events and optimize your peak power and ability to repeat maximum efforts. During this period, training volume generally decreases as intensity increases proportionately.

The **Transition Period** comes after you have reached your goals and have experienced a successful season. While this is the end of one season, it is also the beginning of the next; without proper regeneration between seasons, your fitness from year to year will plateau or regress, rather than progress. The Transition Period is a time of active physical regeneration, unstructured workouts, and decreased volume and intensity.

Regeneration is important throughout your training program. A balance of training stimulus and recovery gradually leads you to peak performance. For a full explanation of periodization, see *The Ultimate Ride*.

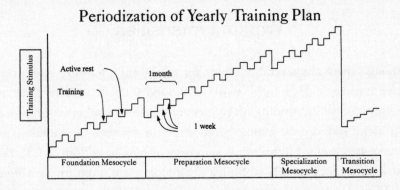

Periodization of Yearly Training Plan

Training Stimulus

Active rest

Training

1 month

1 week

Foundation Mesocycle	Preparation Mesocycle	Specialization Mesocycle	Transition Mesocycle

Overreaching vs. Overtraining

You have to be careful to maintain the delicate balance between work and recovery in order to arrive at your goal event optimally prepared. During periods of high intensity and/or volume, you need to increase your focus on your body and its response to the training load, since these are the times when positive **overreaching** can give way to detrimental **overtraining**. Both are states of fatigue, but one leads to improved performance while the other can bring an early end to your season.

Overreaching is a positive adaptation to training, which often occurs as the result of progressively increasing training loads over a period of two weeks. Signs of overreaching include increased resting heart rate, trouble sleeping, and increased levels of perceived exertion during workouts (regardless of whether or not the workouts are harder or easier). With overreaching, these signs disappear and performance improves after about a week of regeneration.

When signs of overreaching persist and a week of regeneration does not help, you may be facing **overtraining**, which occurs when you push too hard without enough time to recover and adapt to the training stimulus. Signs that you have crossed the line from overreaching to overtraining include: resting heart rate elevated by five to ten beats for more than two days, unexpected weight loss and pronounced fatigue, as well as significant mood and sleep disturbances. These signs are similar to overreaching; however, you are typically not able to recover within four to seven days. In an overtraining situation, it may take four weeks to two months to get your program back on track.

Workout Intensities

Although there are several methods for establishing training intensities, I prefer to use a field test that consists of two short time trials, preferably over the same course. Depending on your circumstances (weather or terrain), the CTS Field Test can be a time-based effort (8 minutes in duration) or a distance-based effort (3 miles). A summary of how to perform a CTS Field Test is given on page 231 (complete instructions are given in *The Ultimate Ride.*) These tests reveal your maximum sustainable heart rate and power output in real-world conditions, making them a practical, accurate, repeatable, and economical means of establishing training intensities from your personal performance data. I recommend a field test every 6–8 weeks throughout the year to ensure your training intensities keep pace with your progress.

When you're using a heart rate monitor or power meter to establish training intensities for specific workouts, it's easy to get the exact heart rate and power numbers confused. This is especially true as your power ranges change in response to training progress. To alleviate this potential problem, record your numbers after each performance test. (See Appendix for the chart to track your CTS Field Test performance.)

Calculating Heart Rate Ranges from the CTS Field Test

To determine your various heart rate ranges from the CTS Field Test data, apply the percentages listed below to the highest average heart rate from your field test. This provides the low number of the range. Next, add 2 to 4 beats to determine the high number of the range.

	Senior (< 35 years)	Master (≥ 35 years)
FoundationMiles™	≤ 89%	≤ 86%
EnduranceMiles™	≤ 91%	≤ 88%
RecoveryMiles™	≤ 70%	≤ 70%
Tempo™	88% (low) + 2–4 beats (high)	87% (low) + 2–4 beats (high)
SteadyState™	92% (low) + 2–4 beats (high)	90% (low) + 2–4 beats (high)
ClimbingRepeats™	95% (low) + 2–4 beats (high)	92% (low) + 2–4 beats (high)

For example, take a senior whose average heart rates during the field test were 183 (effort #1) and 185 (effort #2). The lower limit of her heart rate range for a Tempo™ ride would be: 185 (the higher of the two) × 0.88 = 162.80 rounded to 163 bpm. To generate the heart rate range for Tempo™ workouts, add 2–4 bpm to 163 (we will add four). The Tempo™ heart rate range for this senior athlete becomes 163–167.

I recommend using "heart rate ceilings" during FoundationMiles™(FM) and EnduranceMiles™(EM) rides instead of prescribing lower limits to heart rate. These heart rate ceilings are useful because they provide a specific marker that you should stay under in order to facilitate development of the aerobic energy system. By only providing a ceiling, you have a great deal of freedom, and it is usually in the context of group rides that a ceiling is most appropriate, especially in the Foundation and Preparation Periods of training.

Calculating Power Ranges from Your CTS Field Test Data

To determine your various wattage ranges and ceilings from CTS Field Test data, apply the percentages listed below to the average of the two individual average power outputs from your field test. Unlike the heart rate ranges, cyclists of all ages can use the same percentages to calculate power ranges.

	Low End of Range	High End of Range
FoundationMiles™	40%	67%
EnduranceMiles™	45%	73%
RecoveryMiles™	30%	50%
Tempo™	81%	85%
SteadyState™	86%	90%
ClimbingRepeats™	95%	100%

Recording Workout Intensities

Whether you're using the CTS Field Test and calculations, or you're using another method for determining training intensities, use the table on page 12 to record your heart rate and/or power ranges.

Workout	Date	Power Range	HR Range
Ex: FM		100–160 watts	118–140 bpm
RecoveryMiles™			
FoundationMiles™			
EnduranceMiles™			
Tempo™			
SteadyState™			
ClimbingRepeats™			
Max Effort			
Other Workouts:			

The Role of a Coach

While it is possible to be a successful self-coached athlete, a coach can be a great asset to your training. A coach's role goes well beyond designing your workout schedule. He/she interprets your response to training and evaluates your readiness for upcoming work. In addition, a coach can help you create your long-term goals, develop a nutrition plan, and manage your time more efficiently. Training modifications can be made swiftly so that you, as the athlete, can maintain your focus on your training and have confidence that a professional is closely monitoring your overall progress. For more information on athletic and nutrition coaching, please visit www.trainright.com to check out our complete line of services.

How to Use Your Daily Training Diary

In your training diary, each day of the week has been divided into three parts. The individual sections include baseline data, training data, and personal data. Recording information in each of these sections will allow you to not only track your training progress, but also to see how outside activities affect training and vice versa.

Baseline Data

The first thing you will enter into your daily log will be your baseline data. This information will help you evaluate your body's response to training, especially in relation to your recovery time. Baseline data should remain relatively constant throughout the year; deviations from normal indicate you are having trouble adapting to the training load. This information can be useful on a daily, as well as on a long-term basis. Significant changes in waking weight over a period of two or three days call for modifications in the training load, any time of the year. Over a longer period of time, you can evaluate trends in your improved fitness.

To use this section properly, the information you should record is:

Waking Heart Rate: Your heart rate while lying down, before you get out of bed. To establish a baseline for waking heart rate, you need to record a week's worth of data while you are well rested. During this restful week, your waking heart rate should be relatively consistent (within a few beats) each morning. During your training weeks, it is best to average the week's waking heart rates before deciding to change your training load. Avoid the temptation to make immediate changes to your training schedule based on an anomaly one morning.

Standing Heart Rate: Your heart rate ten seconds after you get out of bed.

Waking Weight: Your weight after you use the bathroom, but before you eat or drink. Your body weight will fluctuate slightly based on hydration state and diet, but large changes from day to day are not normal. Under normal conditions, it is very uncommon for any person to gain or lose two pounds or more of body weight in a two-day (48-hour) period. If you notice weight fluctuations of this magnitude, something is not right.

Sleep: How many hours you have slept, the quality of your sleep (1: horrible to 10: fantastic) and comments to describe your previous night's sleep (restful, interrupted, tossing, etc.).

Mood: The quality of your mood (1: horrible to 10: fantastic), and descriptive adjectives (positive, motivated, stressed, lethargic, etc.).

Training Data

This section is used to record the details of your daily workouts. Over time you will be able to use this information to identify trends in your power output, training load, and other performance markers.

In this section, record the following:

Goal: Your goal for training that day, what you want to accomplish during your workout.

Workout: Your targeted workout for the day, total time prescribed and specific tasks, as well as your actual workout time, distance, cadence, average power, and heart rates. You should also record the information about each individual interval/specific task (time, heart rate, and power).

Notes: Record any other information about your workout that you would like to keep record of (weather, mechanical issues, food intake, etc).

Personal Data

You should use this section to record other significant aspects of your life. If cycling is an integral part of your life, then your life is definitely an integral part of your cycling. This kind of information allows you to get a glimpse as to how your life affects your training and vice versa. Things to consider including are: hours at work or school, hours on your feet during the day, relationship status (spouse, partner, parents, children), financial issues, tests/exams, holidays, etc.

Weekly Summary

At the end of each week, it's good to take a moment to evaluate the quality and quantity of training you completed during the previous seven days. The information in your weekly summaries can show trends more clearly than looking at individual days, and gives you a good opportunity to check your progress against your yearly periodization plan. Recording averages for sleep hours, sleep quality, and mood state can alert you to elevated fatigue levels and perhaps impending illness. We've also added a strength training record to the end of each week.

In addition to recording baseline, training, and personal information each week, you should also write down as many specifics as possible about any competitions or events you participate in. More important than the distance, time, or result are your comments about what went well during the event, and what you can work on for next time. You can record this information in the weekly race records provided at the end of the weekly summary.

How to Use the Appendix

At the end of the daily diary, you will notice a collection of data sheets to fill out. The purpose of your training diary is not only to keep record of your daily information, but also to have a place for you to keep records of weekly, monthly, and yearly data on your training as well as to keep records of races, equipment, etc.

Here is a list of what you will find and how to use it:

- *Test Results:* Record information from any tests you perform throughout the year (CTS Field Test, LT test, VO_{2max} test, body composition. For a complete rundown of CTS tests, consult *The Ultimate Ride*).
- *Event Results:* Record the basic data of your events here for an easy glimpse across your season.
- *Do-It-Yourself Graphs:* Use these tables to plot information gathered during the course of individual months. For instance, you could use one of these graphs to see how your waking weight changed during the course of February. Similarly, you could use them to build a graphic representation of your training hours for the month.
- *Bike Fit:* Record all of your bike measurements and any changes you make to your equipment. This comes in extremely handy when you travel with your bike or when you have to purchase and install new parts.
- *Equipment Log:* Record the dates of any purchases or repairs.
- *Pre-Event Checklist:* Use this checklist to make sure you don't forget something important when you travel to your events. Remember, al-

ways carry your pedals, shoes, and helmet in your carry-on baggage when you fly. Those are the items that are hardest to borrow if your luggage gets lost.

- *Contacts:* Use this section to keep important phone numbers, email addresses, and websites handy.

Before getting started, take a moment to lay your season out in front of you. Use the following chart to lay out the foundation of your training plan. When do your events occur? What should be happening in July? What are your goals on a weekly basis? What workouts do you plan to do? This chart will help you stay on track and ultimately reach your goal.

Your Year-Long Training Plan

Season/Long-Term Goal: _____

Target Date: _____ Start Date: _____

Week	Date	Goal	Training Period	Hours	Workouts	Weights	Tests	Races
	4/4–4/10	Aerobic Development	Foundation	10	FM, FP, RM, PS	yes		Red Park Cyclo-cross
	4/11–4/17	Aerobic Development and Leg Speed	Foundation	12	FM, FP, RM, S, RS	yes	Field	
1								
2								
3								
4								
5								
6								
7								
8								
9								
10								
11								
12								
13								
14								
15								
16								
17								
18								
19								
20								
21								

Part 2:

The Training Diary

Week # _____ Goal: _____

Monday ■ Date: ___/___/___

Waking Heart Rate _____

Standing Heart Rate _____

Waking Weight _____ Hours of Sleep _____

Quality of Sleep   1 2 3 4 5 6 7 8 9 10

Mood State   1 2 3 4 5 6 7 8 9 10

Goal _____

Workout _____

Specific Task _____

Actual Workout Time _____

Distance _____ Cadence _____

Average Heart Rate _____ Power _____

Interval 1: TIME _____ HR _____ P _____

Interval 2: TIME _____ HR _____ P _____

Interval 3: TIME _____ HR _____ P _____

Interval 4: TIME _____ HR _____ P _____

Interval 5: TIME _____ HR _____ P _____

Workout Notes _____

Personal Notes _____

Tuesday ■ Date: ___/___/___

Waking Heart Rate _____

Standing Heart Rate _____

Waking Weight _____ Hours of Sleep _____

Quality of Sleep   1 2 3 4 5 6 7 8 9 10

Mood State   1 2 3 4 5 6 7 8 9 10

Goal _____

Workout _____

Specific Task _____

Actual Workout Time _____

Distance _____ Cadence _____

Average Heart Rate _____ Power _____

Interval 1: TIME _____ HR _____ P _____

Interval 2: TIME _____ HR _____ P _____

Interval 3: TIME _____ HR _____ P _____

Interval 4: TIME _____ HR _____ P _____

Interval 5: TIME _____ HR _____ P _____

Workout Notes _____

Personal Notes _____

Wednesday ■ Date: ___/___/___

Waking Heart Rate _____

Standing Heart Rate _____

Waking Weight _____ Hours of Sleep _____

Quality of Sleep   1 2 3 4 5 6 7 8 9 10

Mood State   1 2 3 4 5 6 7 8 9 10

Goal _____

Workout _____

Specific Task _____

Actual Workout Time _____

Distance _____ Cadence _____

Average Heart Rate _____ Power _____

Interval 1: TIME _____ HR _____ P _____

Interval 2: TIME _____ HR _____ P _____

Interval 3: TIME _____ HR _____ P _____

Interval 4: TIME _____ HR _____ P _____

Interval 5: TIME _____ HR _____ P _____

Workout Notes _____

Personal Notes _____

Thursday ■ Date: ___/___/___

Waking Heart Rate _____

Standing Heart Rate _____

Waking Weight _____ Hours of Sleep _____

Quality of Sleep 1 2 3 4 5 6 7 8 9 10

Mood State 1 2 3 4 5 6 7 8 9 10

Goal _____

Workout _____

Specific Task _____

Actual Workout Time _____

Distance _____ Cadence _____

Average Heart Rate _____ Power _____

Interval 1: TIME _____ HR _____ P _____

Interval 2: TIME _____ HR _____ P _____

Interval 3: TIME _____ HR _____ P _____

Interval 4: TIME _____ HR _____ P _____

Interval 5: TIME _____ HR _____ P _____

Workout Notes _____

Personal Notes _____

Friday ■ Date: ___/___/___

Waking Heart Rate _____

Standing Heart Rate _____

Waking Weight _____ Hours of Sleep _____

Quality of Sleep 1 2 3 4 5 6 7 8 9 10

Mood State 1 2 3 4 5 6 7 8 9 10

Goal _____

Workout _____

Specific Task _____

Actual Workout Time _____

Distance _____ Cadence _____

Average Heart Rate _____ Power _____

Interval 1: TIME _____ HR _____ P _____

Interval 2: TIME _____ HR _____ P _____

Interval 3: TIME _____ HR _____ P _____

Interval 4: TIME _____ HR _____ P _____

Interval 5: TIME _____ HR _____ P _____

Workout Notes _____

Personal Notes _____

Saturday ■ Date: ___/___/___

Waking Heart Rate _____

Standing Heart Rate _____

Waking Weight _____ Hours of Sleep _____

Quality of Sleep 1 2 3 4 5 6 7 8 9 10

Mood State 1 2 3 4 5 6 7 8 9 10

Goal _____

Workout _____

Specific Task _____

Actual Workout Time _____

Distance _____ Cadence _____

Average Heart Rate _____ Power _____

Interval 1: TIME _____ HR _____ P _____

Interval 2: TIME _____ HR _____ P _____

Interval 3: TIME _____ HR _____ P _____

Interval 4: TIME _____ HR _____ P _____

Interval 5: TIME _____ HR _____ P _____

Workout Notes _____

Personal Notes _____

| Week # |

Sunday ■ Date: ___ / ___ / ___

Waking Heart Rate _____

Standing Heart Rate _____

Waking Weight _____ Hours of Sleep _____

Quality of Sleep 1 2 3 4 5 6 7 8 9 10

Mood State 1 2 3 4 5 6 7 8 9 10

Goal _____

Workout _____

Specific Task _____

Actual Workout Time _____

Distance _____ Cadence _____

Average Heart Rate _____ Power _____

Interval 1: TIME _____ HR _____ P _____

Interval 2: TIME _____ HR _____ P _____

Interval 3: TIME _____ HR _____ P _____

Interval 4: TIME _____ HR _____ P _____

Interval 5: TIME _____ HR _____ P _____

Workout Notes _____

Personal Notes _____

Weekly Summary

Hours of Cycling: _____ Year-to-Date: _____

Miles/Kilometers: _____ Year-to-Date: _____

Hours of Strength Training: _____ Year-to-Date: _____

Hours of Other Activities: _____ Year-to-Date: _____

_____ Year-to-Date: _____

_____ Year-to-Date: _____

_____ Year-to-Date: _____

Total Training Hours: _____ Year-to-Date: _____

Number of Workouts Planned: _____

Number of Workouts Completed: ____

Average Hours of Sleep: _____

Average Quality of Sleep: _____

Average Mood State: _____

Time Spent in Heart Rate/Power Ranges:

CTS RANGES	TIME	CTS RANGES	TIME	OTHER WORKOUTS	TIME
RecoveryMiles™		SteadyState™			
FoundationMiles™		ClimbingRepeats™			
EnduranceMiles™		Max Effort			
Tempo™					

Personal Notes: _____

Race Results

Race #1 _____ Date: ___ / ___ / ___

Time _____ Distance _____

Goal _____

Result _____

Average Heart Rate _____ Power _____

Food/Fluid Intake _____

Personal Notes _____

_____

_____

Race #2 _____ Date: ___ / ___ / ___

Time _____ Distance _____

Goal _____

Result _____

Average Heart Rate _____ Power _____

Food/Fluid Intake _____

Personal Notes _____

_____

_____

Week # _____

Weekly Strength Training Record

Exercise	Date:						Date:						Date:					
	SET 1		SET 2		SET 3		SET 1		SET 2		SET 3		SET 1		SET 2		SET 3	
	lbs.	reps	lbs.	reps	lbs.	reps	lbs.	reps	lbs.	reps	lbs.	reps	lbs.	reps	lbs.	reps	lbs.	reps

Week # _____   Goal: _____

Monday ■ Date: ___ / ___ / ___

Waking Heart Rate _____

Standing Heart Rate _____

Waking Weight _____ Hours of Sleep _____

Quality of Sleep 1 2 3 4 5 6 7 8 9 10

Mood State 1 2 3 4 5 6 7 8 9 10

Goal _____

Workout _____

Specific Task _____

Actual Workout Time _____

Distance _____ Cadence _____

Average Heart Rate _____ Power _____

Interval 1: TIME _____ HR _____ P _____

Interval 2: TIME _____ HR _____ P _____

Interval 3: TIME _____ HR _____ P _____

Interval 4: TIME _____ HR _____ P _____

Interval 5: TIME _____ HR _____ P _____

Workout Notes _____

Personal Notes _____

Tuesday ■ Date: ___ / ___ / ___

Waking Heart Rate _____

Standing Heart Rate _____

Waking Weight _____ Hours of Sleep _____

Quality of Sleep 1 2 3 4 5 6 7 8 9 10

Mood State 1 2 3 4 5 6 7 8 9 10

Goal _____

Workout _____

Specific Task _____

Actual Workout Time _____

Distance _____ Cadence _____

Average Heart Rate _____ Power _____

Interval 1: TIME _____ HR _____ P _____

Interval 2: TIME _____ HR _____ P _____

Interval 3: TIME _____ HR _____ P _____

Interval 4: TIME _____ HR _____ P _____

Interval 5: TIME _____ HR _____ P _____

Workout Notes _____

Personal Notes _____

Wednesday ■ Date: ___ / ___ / ___

Waking Heart Rate _____

Standing Heart Rate _____

Waking Weight _____ Hours of Sleep _____

Quality of Sleep 1 2 3 4 5 6 7 8 9 10

Mood State 1 2 3 4 5 6 7 8 9 10

Goal _____

Workout _____

Specific Task _____

Actual Workout Time _____

Distance _____ Cadence _____

Average Heart Rate _____ Power _____

Interval 1: TIME _____ HR _____ P _____

Interval 2: TIME _____ HR _____ P _____

Interval 3: TIME _____ HR _____ P _____

Interval 4: TIME _____ HR _____ P _____

Interval 5: TIME _____ HR _____ P _____

Workout Notes _____

Personal Notes _____

Thursday ■ Date: ___ / ___ / ___

Waking Heart Rate ___
Standing Heart Rate ___
Waking Weight ___ Hours of Sleep ___
Quality of Sleep   1 2 3 4 5 6 7 8 9 10

Mood State   1 2 3 4 5 6 7 8 9 10

Goal ___
Workout ___
Specific Task ___
Actual Workout Time ___
Distance ___ Cadence ___
Average Heart Rate ___ Power ___

Interval 1: TIME ___ HR ___ P ___
Interval 2: TIME ___ HR ___ P ___
Interval 3: TIME ___ HR ___ P ___
Interval 4: TIME ___ HR ___ P ___
Interval 5: TIME ___ HR ___ P ___

Workout Notes ___

Personal Notes ___

Friday ■ Date: ___ / ___ / ___

Waking Heart Rate ___
Standing Heart Rate ___
Waking Weight ___ Hours of Sleep ___
Quality of Sleep   1 2 3 4 5 6 7 8 9 10

Mood State   1 2 3 4 5 6 7 8 9 10

Goal ___
Workout ___
Specific Task ___
Actual Workout Time ___
Distance ___ Cadence ___
Average Heart Rate ___ Power ___

Interval 1: TIME ___ HR ___ P ___
Interval 2: TIME ___ HR ___ P ___
Interval 3: TIME ___ HR ___ P ___
Interval 4: TIME ___ HR ___ P ___
Interval 5: TIME ___ HR ___ P ___

Workout Notes ___

Personal Notes ___

Saturday ■ Date: ___ / ___ / ___

Waking Heart Rate ___
Standing Heart Rate ___
Waking Weight ___ Hours of Sleep ___
Quality of Sleep   1 2 3 4 5 6 7 8 9 10

Mood State   1 2 3 4 5 6 7 8 9 10

Goal ___
Workout ___
Specific Task ___
Actual Workout Time ___
Distance ___ Cadence ___
Average Heart Rate ___ Power ___

Interval 1: TIME ___ HR ___ P ___
Interval 2: TIME ___ HR ___ P ___
Interval 3: TIME ___ HR ___ P ___
Interval 4: TIME ___ HR ___ P ___
Interval 5: TIME ___ HR ___ P ___

Workout Notes ___

Personal Notes ___

Week #

Sunday ■ Date: ___ / ___ / ___

Waking Heart Rate ___

Standing Heart Rate ___

Waking Weight ___ Hours of Sleep ___

Quality of Sleep 1 2 3 4 5 6 7 8 9 10

Mood State 1 2 3 4 5 6 7 8 9 10

Goal ___

Workout ___

Specific Task ___

Actual Workout Time ___

Distance ___ Cadence ___

Average Heart Rate ___ Power ___

Interval 1: TIME ___ HR ___ P ___
Interval 2: TIME ___ HR ___ P ___
Interval 3: TIME ___ HR ___ P ___
Interval 4: TIME ___ HR ___ P ___
Interval 5: TIME ___ HR ___ P ___

Workout Notes ___

Personal Notes ___

Weekly Summary

Hours of Cycling: ___ Year-to-Date: ___

Miles/Kilometers: ___ Year-to-Date: ___

Hours of Strength Training: ___ Year-to-Date: ___

Hours of Other Activities: ___

___ Year-to-Date: ___

___ Year-to-Date: ___

___ Year-to-Date: ___

___ Year-to-Date: ___

Total Training Hours: ___

Number of Workouts Planned: ___

Number of Workouts Completed: ___

Average Hours of Sleep: ___

Average Quality of Sleep: ___

Average Mood State: ___

Time Spent in Heart Rate/Power Ranges:

CTS RANGES	TIME	CTS RANGES	TIME	OTHER WORKOUTS	TIME
RecoveryMiles™	___	SteadyState™	___	___	___
FoundationMiles™	___	ClimbingRepeats™	___	___	___
EnduranceMiles™	___	Max Effort	___	___	___
Tempo™	___			___	___

Personal Notes: ___

Weekly Strength Training Record

Exercise	Date:						Date:						Date:					
	SET 1		SET 2		SET 3		SET 1		SET 2		SET 3		SET 1		SET 2		SET 3	
	lbs.	reps	lbs.	reps	lbs.	reps	lbs.	reps	lbs.	reps	lbs.	reps	lbs.	reps	lbs.	reps	lbs.	reps

Race Results

Race #1 _____ Date: ___/___/___

Time _____ Distance _____

Goal _____

Result _____

Average Heart Rate _____ Power _____

Food/Fluid Intake _____

Personal Notes _____

_____

_____

_____

Race #2 _____ Date: ___/___/___

Time _____ Distance _____

Goal _____

Result _____

Average Heart Rate _____ Power _____

Food/Fluid Intake _____

Personal Notes _____

_____

_____

_____

| Week # | | Goal: |

Monday ■ Date: ___ / ___ / ___

Waking Heart Rate

Standing Heart Rate

Waking Weight _____ Hours of Sleep _____

Quality of Sleep 1 2 3 4 5 6 7 8 9 10

Mood State 1 2 3 4 5 6 7 8 9 10

Goal

Workout

Specific Task

Actual Workout Time

Distance _____ Cadence _____ Power _____

Average Heart Rate _____ Power _____

Interval 1: TIME _____ HR _____ P _____
Interval 2: TIME _____ HR _____ P _____
Interval 3: TIME _____ HR _____ P _____
Interval 4: TIME _____ HR _____ P _____
Interval 5: TIME _____ HR _____ P _____

Workout Notes

Personal Notes

Tuesday ■ Date: ___ / ___ / ___

Waking Heart Rate

Standing Heart Rate

Waking Weight _____ Hours of Sleep _____

Quality of Sleep 1 2 3 4 5 6 7 8 9 10

Mood State 1 2 3 4 5 6 7 8 9 10

Goal

Workout

Specific Task

Actual Workout Time

Distance _____ Cadence _____ Power _____

Average Heart Rate _____ Power _____

Interval 1: TIME _____ HR _____ P _____
Interval 2: TIME _____ HR _____ P _____
Interval 3: TIME _____ HR _____ P _____
Interval 4: TIME _____ HR _____ P _____
Interval 5: TIME _____ HR _____ P _____

Workout Notes

Personal Notes

Wednesday ■ Date: ___ / ___ / ___

Waking Heart Rate

Standing Heart Rate

Waking Weight _____ Hours of Sleep _____

Quality of Sleep 1 2 3 4 5 6 7 8 9 10

Mood State 1 2 3 4 5 6 7 8 9 10

Goal

Workout

Specific Task

Actual Workout Time

Distance _____ Cadence _____ Power _____

Average Heart Rate _____ Power _____

Interval 1: TIME _____ HR _____ P _____
Interval 2: TIME _____ HR _____ P _____
Interval 3: TIME _____ HR _____ P _____
Interval 4: TIME _____ HR _____ P _____
Interval 5: TIME _____ HR _____ P _____

Workout Notes

Personal Notes

Thursday ■ Date: ___ / ___ / ___

Waking Heart Rate _____

Standing Heart Rate _____

Waking Weight _____ Hours of Sleep _____

Quality of Sleep 1 2 3 4 5 6 7 8 9 10

Mood State 1 2 3 4 5 6 7 8 9 10

Goal _____

Workout _____

Specific Task _____

Actual Workout Time _____

Distance _____ Cadence _____

Average Heart Rate _____ Power _____

Interval 1: TIME _____ HR _____ P. _____

Interval 2: TIME _____ HR _____ P. _____

Interval 3: TIME _____ HR _____ P. _____

Interval 4: TIME _____ HR _____ P. _____

Interval 5: TIME _____ HR _____ P. _____

Workout Notes _____

Personal Notes _____

Friday ■ Date: ___ / ___ / ___

Waking Heart Rate _____

Standing Heart Rate _____

Waking Weight _____ Hours of Sleep _____

Quality of Sleep 1 2 3 4 5 6 7 8 9 10

Mood State 1 2 3 4 5 6 7 8 9 10

Goal _____

Workout _____

Specific Task _____

Actual Workout Time _____

Distance _____ Cadence _____

Average Heart Rate _____ Power _____

Interval 1: TIME _____ HR _____ P. _____

Interval 2: TIME _____ HR _____ P. _____

Interval 3: TIME _____ HR _____ P. _____

Interval 4: TIME _____ HR _____ P. _____

Interval 5: TIME _____ HR _____ P. _____

Workout Notes _____

Personal Notes _____

Saturday ■ Date: ___ / ___ / ___

Waking Heart Rate _____

Standing Heart Rate _____

Waking Weight _____ Hours of Sleep _____

Quality of Sleep 1 2 3 4 5 6 7 8 9 10

Mood State 1 2 3 4 5 6 7 8 9 10

Goal _____

Workout _____

Specific Task _____

Actual Workout Time _____

Distance _____ Cadence _____

Average Heart Rate _____ Power _____

Interval 1: TIME _____ HR _____ P. _____

Interval 2: TIME _____ HR _____ P. _____

Interval 3: TIME _____ HR _____ P. _____

Interval 4: TIME _____ HR _____ P. _____

Interval 5: TIME _____ HR _____ P. _____

Workout Notes _____

Personal Notes _____

Week #

Sunday ■ Date: ___ / ___ / ___

Waking Heart Rate ___

Standing Heart Rate ___

Waking Weight ___ Hours of Sleep ___

Quality of Sleep   1 2 3 4 5 6 7 8 9 10

Mood State   1 2 3 4 5 6 7 8 9 10

Goal ___

Workout ___

Specific Task ___

Actual Workout Time ___

Distance ___ Cadence ___

Average Heart Rate ___ Power ___

Interval 1: TIME ___ HR ___ P ___

Interval 2: TIME ___ HR ___ P ___

Interval 3: TIME ___ HR ___ P ___

Interval 4: TIME ___ HR ___ P ___

Interval 5: TIME ___ HR ___ P ___

Workout Notes ___

Personal Notes ___

Weekly Summary

Hours of Cycling: ___ Year-to-Date: ___

Miles/Kilometers: ___ Year-to-Date: ___

Hours of Strength Training: ___ Year-to-Date: ___

Hours of Other Activities: ___

___ Year-to-Date: ___

___ Year-to-Date: ___

___ Year-to-Date: ___

Total Training Hours: ___ Year-to-Date: ___

Number of Workouts Planned: ___

Number of Workouts Completed: ___

Average Hours of Sleep: ___

Average Quality of Sleep: ___

Average Mood State: ___

Time Spent in Heart Rate/Power Ranges:

CTS RANGES	TIME	CTS RANGES	TIME	OTHER WORKOUTS	TIME
RecoveryMiles™		SteadyState™			
FoundationMiles™		ClimbingRepeats™			
EnduranceMiles™		Max Effort			
Tempo™					

Personal Notes: ___

Weekly Strength Training Record

Race Results

Race #1 _____ Date: __ / __ / __

Time _____ Distance _____

Goal _____

Result _____

Average Heart Rate _____ Power _____

Food/Fluid Intake _____

Personal Notes _____

_____

_____

Race #2 _____ Date: __ / __ / __

Time _____ Distance _____

Goal _____

Result _____

Average Heart Rate _____ Power _____

Food/Fluid Intake _____

Personal Notes _____

_____

_____

Exercise	Date:			Date:			Date:		
	SET 1 lbs. / reps	SET 2 lbs. / reps	SET 3 lbs. / reps	SET 1 lbs. / reps	SET 2 lbs. / reps	SET 3 lbs. / reps	SET 1 lbs. / reps	SET 2 lbs. / reps	SET 3 lbs. / reps

Week #		Goal:

Monday ■ Date: ___ / ___ / ___

Waking Heart Rate _____

Standing Heart Rate _____

Waking Weight _____ Hours of Sleep _____

Quality of Sleep   1 2 3 4 5 6 7 8 9 10

Mood State   1 2 3 4 5 6 7 8 9 10

Goal _____

Workout _____

Specific Task _____

Actual Workout Time _____

Distance _____ Cadence _____

Average Heart Rate _____ Power _____

Interval 1: TIME _____ HR _____ P _____

Interval 2: TIME _____ HR _____ P _____

Interval 3: TIME _____ HR _____ P _____

Interval 4: TIME _____ HR _____ P _____

Interval 5: TIME _____ HR _____ P _____

Workout Notes _____

Personal Notes _____

Tuesday ■ Date: ___ / ___ / ___

Waking Heart Rate _____

Standing Heart Rate _____

Waking Weight _____ Hours of Sleep _____

Quality of Sleep   1 2 3 4 5 6 7 8 9 10

Mood State   1 2 3 4 5 6 7 8 9 10

Goal _____

Workout _____

Specific Task _____

Actual Workout Time _____

Distance _____ Cadence _____

Average Heart Rate _____ Power _____

Interval 1: TIME _____ HR _____ P _____

Interval 2: TIME _____ HR _____ P _____

Interval 3: TIME _____ HR _____ P _____

Interval 4: TIME _____ HR _____ P _____

Interval 5: TIME _____ HR _____ P _____

Workout Notes _____

Personal Notes _____

Wednesday ■ Date: ___ / ___ / ___

Waking Heart Rate _____

Standing Heart Rate _____

Waking Weight _____ Hours of Sleep _____

Quality of Sleep   1 2 3 4 5 6 7 8 9 10

Mood State   1 2 3 4 5 6 7 8 9 10

Goal _____

Workout _____

Specific Task _____

Actual Workout Time _____

Distance _____ Cadence _____

Average Heart Rate _____ Power _____

Interval 1: TIME _____ HR _____ P _____

Interval 2: TIME _____ HR _____ P _____

Interval 3: TIME _____ HR _____ P _____

Interval 4: TIME _____ HR _____ P _____

Interval 5: TIME _____ HR _____ P _____

Workout Notes _____

Personal Notes _____

Thursday ■ Date: ___/___/___

Waking Heart Rate _____

Standing Heart Rate _____

Waking Weight _____ Hours of Sleep _____

Quality of Sleep   1 2 3 4 5 6 7 8 9 10

Mood State   1 2 3 4 5 6 7 8 9 10

Goal _____

Workout _____

Specific Task _____

Actual Workout Time _____

Distance _____ Cadence _____

Average Heart Rate _____ Power _____

Interval 1: TIME _____ HR _____ P _____
Interval 2: TIME _____ HR _____ P _____
Interval 3: TIME _____ HR _____ P _____
Interval 4: TIME _____ HR _____ P _____
Interval 5: TIME _____ HR _____ P _____

Workout Notes _____

Personal Notes _____

Friday ■ Date: ___/___/___

Waking Heart Rate _____

Standing Heart Rate _____

Waking Weight _____ Hours of Sleep _____

Quality of Sleep   1 2 3 4 5 6 7 8 9 10

Mood State   1 2 3 4 5 6 7 8 9 10

Goal _____

Workout _____

Specific Task _____

Actual Workout Time _____

Distance _____ Cadence _____

Average Heart Rate _____ Power _____

Interval 1: TIME _____ HR _____ P _____
Interval 2: TIME _____ HR _____ P _____
Interval 3: TIME _____ HR _____ P _____
Interval 4: TIME _____ HR _____ P _____
Interval 5: TIME _____ HR _____ P _____

Workout Notes _____

Personal Notes _____

Saturday ■ Date: ___/___/___

Waking Heart Rate _____

Standing Heart Rate _____

Waking Weight _____ Hours of Sleep _____

Quality of Sleep   1 2 3 4 5 6 7 8 9 10

Mood State   1 2 3 4 5 6 7 8 9 10

Goal _____

Workout _____

Specific Task _____

Actual Workout Time _____

Distance _____ Cadence _____

Average Heart Rate _____ Power _____

Interval 1: TIME _____ HR _____ P _____
Interval 2: TIME _____ HR _____ P _____
Interval 3: TIME _____ HR _____ P _____
Interval 4: TIME _____ HR _____ P _____
Interval 5: TIME _____ HR _____ P _____

Workout Notes _____

Personal Notes _____

Week #

Sunday ■ Date: ___ / ___ / ___

Waking Heart Rate _____

Standing Heart Rate _____

Waking Weight _____ Hours of Sleep _____

Quality of Sleep 1 2 3 4 5 6 7 8 9 10

Mood State 1 2 3 4 5 6 7 8 9 10

Goal _____

Workout _____

Specific Task _____

Actual Workout Time _____

Distance _____ Cadence _____

Average Heart Rate _____ Power _____

Interval 1: TIME _____ HR _____ P _____
Interval 2: TIME _____ HR _____ P _____
Interval 3: TIME _____ HR _____ P _____
Interval 4: TIME _____ HR _____ P _____
Interval 5: TIME _____ HR _____ P _____

Workout Notes _____

Personal Notes _____

Weekly Summary

Hours of Cycling: _____ Year-to-Date: _____

Miles/Kilometers: _____ Year-to-Date: _____

Hours of Strength Training: _____ Year-to-Date: _____

Hours of Other Activities: _____ Year-to-Date: _____

_____ Year-to-Date: _____

_____ Year-to-Date: _____

_____ Year-to-Date: _____

_____ Year-to-Date: _____

Total Training Hours: _____

Number of Workouts Planned: _____

Number of Workouts Completed: _____

Average Hours of Sleep: _____

Average Quality of Sleep: _____

Average Mood State: _____

Time Spent in Heart Rate/Power Ranges:

CTS RANGES	TIME	CTS RANGES	TIME	OTHER WORKOUTS	TIME
RecoveryMiles™		SteadyState™			
FoundationMiles™		ClimbingRepeats™			
EnduranceMiles™		Max Effort			
Tempo™					

Personal Notes: _____

| 34 |

Weekly Strength Training Record

Race Results

Race #1 _____ Date: ___ / ___ / ___

Time _____ Distance _____

Goal _____

Result _____

Average Heart Rate _____ Power _____

Food/Fluid Intake _____

Personal Notes _____

Race #2 _____ Date: ___ / ___ / ___

Time _____ Distance _____

Goal _____

Result _____

Average Heart Rate _____ Power _____

Food/Fluid Intake _____

Personal Notes _____

Exercise	Date:						Date:						Date:					
	SET 1		SET 2		SET 3		SET 1		SET 2		SET 3		SET 1		SET 2		SET 3	
	lbs.	reps	lbs.	reps	lbs.	reps	lbs.	reps	lbs.	reps	lbs.	reps	lbs.	reps	lbs.	reps	lbs.	reps

Week # _____   Goal: _____

Monday ▪ Date: ___ / ___ / ___

Waking Heart Rate _____

Standing Heart Rate _____

Waking Weight _____ Hours of Sleep _____

Quality of Sleep 1 2 3 4 5 6 7 8 9 10

Mood State 1 2 3 4 5 6 7 8 9 10

Goal _____

Workout _____

Specific Task _____

Actual Workout Time _____

Distance _____ Cadence _____

Average Heart Rate _____ Power _____

Interval 1: TIME _____ HR _____ P _____
Interval 2: TIME _____ HR _____ P _____
Interval 3: TIME _____ HR _____ P _____
Interval 4: TIME _____ HR _____ P _____
Interval 5: TIME _____ HR _____ P _____

Workout Notes _____

Personal Notes _____

Tuesday ▪ Date: ___ / ___ / ___

Waking Heart Rate _____

Standing Heart Rate _____

Waking Weight _____ Hours of Sleep _____

Quality of Sleep 1 2 3 4 5 6 7 8 9 10

Mood State 1 2 3 4 5 6 7 8 9 10

Goal _____

Workout _____

Specific Task _____

Actual Workout Time _____

Distance _____ Cadence _____

Average Heart Rate _____ Power _____

Interval 1: TIME _____ HR _____ P _____
Interval 2: TIME _____ HR _____ P _____
Interval 3: TIME _____ HR _____ P _____
Interval 4: TIME _____ HR _____ P _____
Interval 5: TIME _____ HR _____ P _____

Workout Notes _____

Personal Notes _____

Wednesday ▪ Date: ___ / ___ / ___

Waking Heart Rate _____

Standing Heart Rate _____

Waking Weight _____ Hours of Sleep _____

Quality of Sleep 1 2 3 4 5 6 7 8 9 10

Mood State 1 2 3 4 5 6 7 8 9 10

Goal _____

Workout _____

Specific Task _____

Actual Workout Time _____

Distance _____ Cadence _____

Average Heart Rate _____ Power _____

Interval 1: TIME _____ HR _____ P _____
Interval 2: TIME _____ HR _____ P _____
Interval 3: TIME _____ HR _____ P _____
Interval 4: TIME _____ HR _____ P _____
Interval 5: TIME _____ HR _____ P _____

Workout Notes _____

Personal Notes _____

Week #

Thursday ■ Date: ___ / ___ / ___

Waking Heart Rate _____

Standing Heart Rate _____

Waking Weight _____ Hours of Sleep _____

Quality of Sleep 1 2 3 4 5 6 7 8 9 10

Mood State 1 2 3 4 5 6 7 8 9 10

Goal _____

Workout _____

Specific Task _____

Actual Workout Time _____

Distance _____ Cadence _____

Average Heart Rate _____ Power _____

Interval 1:	TIME _____	HR _____	P _____
Interval 2:	TIME _____	HR _____	P _____
Interval 3:	TIME _____	HR _____	P _____
Interval 4:	TIME _____	HR _____	P _____
Interval 5:	TIME _____	HR _____	P _____

Workout Notes _____

Personal Notes _____

Friday ■ Date: ___ / ___ / ___

Waking Heart Rate _____

Standing Heart Rate _____

Waking Weight _____ Hours of Sleep _____

Quality of Sleep 1 2 3 4 5 6 7 8 9 10

Mood State 1 2 3 4 5 6 7 8 9 10

Goal _____

Workout _____

Specific Task _____

Actual Workout Time _____

Distance _____ Cadence _____

Average Heart Rate _____ Power _____

Interval 1:	TIME _____	HR _____	P _____
Interval 2:	TIME _____	HR _____	P _____
Interval 3:	TIME _____	HR _____	P _____
Interval 4:	TIME _____	HR _____	P _____
Interval 5:	TIME _____	HR _____	P _____

Workout Notes _____

Personal Notes _____

Saturday ■ Date: ___ / ___ / ___

Waking Heart Rate _____

Standing Heart Rate _____

Waking Weight _____ Hours of Sleep _____

Quality of Sleep 1 2 3 4 5 6 7 8 9 10

Mood State 1 2 3 4 5 6 7 8 9 10

Goal _____

Workout _____

Specific Task _____

Actual Workout Time _____

Distance _____ Cadence _____

Average Heart Rate _____ Power _____

Interval 1:	TIME _____	HR _____	P _____
Interval 2:	TIME _____	HR _____	P _____
Interval 3:	TIME _____	HR _____	P _____
Interval 4:	TIME _____	HR _____	P _____
Interval 5:	TIME _____	HR _____	P _____

Workout Notes _____

Personal Notes _____

Week #

Sunday ■ Date: ___ / ___ / ___

Waking Heart Rate _____

Standing Heart Rate _____

Waking Weight _____ Hours of Sleep _____

Quality of Sleep 1 2 3 4 5 6 7 8 9 10

Mood State 1 2 3 4 5 6 7 8 9 10

Goal _____

Workout _____

Specific Task _____

Actual Workout Time _____

Distance _____ Cadence _____

Average Heart Rate _____ Power _____

Interval 1:	TIME ____	HR ____	P ____
Interval 2:	TIME ____	HR ____	P ____
Interval 3:	TIME ____	HR ____	P ____
Interval 4:	TIME ____	HR ____	P ____
Interval 5:	TIME ____	HR ____	P ____

Workout Notes _____

Personal Notes _____

Weekly Summary

Hours of Cycling: _____ Year-to-Date: _____

Miles/Kilometers: _____ Year-to-Date: _____

Hours of Strength Training: _____ Year-to-Date: _____

Hours of Other Activities: _____ Year-to-Date: _____

_____ Year-to-Date: _____

_____ Year-to-Date: _____

_____ Year-to-Date: _____

Total Training Hours: _____

Number of Workouts Planned: _____

Number of Workouts Completed: _____

Average Hours of Sleep: _____

Average Quality of Sleep: _____

Average Mood State: _____

Time Spent in Heart Rate/Power Ranges:

CTS RANGES	TIME	CTS RANGES	TIME	OTHER WORKOUTS	TIME
RecoveryMiles™		SteadyState™			
FoundationMiles™		ClimbingRepeats™			
EnduranceMiles™		Max Effort			
Tempo™					

Personal Notes: _____

Weekly Strength Training Record

Exercise	Date:						Date:						Date:					
	SET 1		SET 2		SET 3		SET 1		SET 2		SET 3		SET 1		SET 2		SET 3	
	lbs.	reps	lbs.	reps	lbs.	reps	lbs.	reps	lbs.	reps	lbs.	reps	lbs.	reps	lbs.	reps	lbs.	reps

Race Results

Race #1 _____ Date: ___ / ___ / ___

Time _____ Distance _____

Goal _____

Result _____

Average Heart Rate _____ Power _____

Food/Fluid Intake _____

Personal Notes _____

Race #2 _____ Date: ___ / ___ / ___

Time _____ Distance _____

Goal _____

Result _____

Average Heart Rate _____ Power _____

Food/Fluid Intake _____

Personal Notes _____

Week # _____ Goal: _____

Monday ■ Date: ___ / ___ / ___

Waking Heart Rate _____

Standing Heart Rate _____

Waking Weight _____ Hours of Sleep _____

Quality of Sleep 1 2 3 4 5 6 7 8 9 10

Mood State 1 2 3 4 5 6 7 8 9 10

Goal _____

Workout _____

Specific Task _____

Actual Workout Time _____

Distance _____ Cadence _____

Average Heart Rate _____ Power _____

Interval 1: TIME _____ HR _____ P _____
Interval 2: TIME _____ HR _____ P _____
Interval 3: TIME _____ HR _____ P _____
Interval 4: TIME _____ HR _____ P _____
Interval 5: TIME _____ HR _____ P _____

Workout Notes _____

Personal Notes _____

Tuesday ■ Date: ___ / ___ / ___

Waking Heart Rate _____

Standing Heart Rate _____

Waking Weight _____ Hours of Sleep _____

Quality of Sleep 1 2 3 4 5 6 7 8 9 10

Mood State 1 2 3 4 5 6 7 8 9 10

Goal _____

Workout _____

Specific Task _____

Actual Workout Time _____

Distance _____ Cadence _____

Average Heart Rate _____ Power _____

Interval 1: TIME _____ HR _____ P _____
Interval 2: TIME _____ HR _____ P _____
Interval 3: TIME _____ HR _____ P _____
Interval 4: TIME _____ HR _____ P _____
Interval 5: TIME _____ HR _____ P _____

Workout Notes _____

Personal Notes _____

Wednesday ■ Date: ___ / ___ / ___

Waking Heart Rate _____

Standing Heart Rate _____

Waking Weight _____ Hours of Sleep _____

Quality of Sleep 1 2 3 4 5 6 7 8 9 10

Mood State 1 2 3 4 5 6 7 8 9 10

Goal _____

Workout _____

Specific Task _____

Actual Workout Time _____

Distance _____ Cadence _____

Average Heart Rate _____ Power _____

Interval 1: TIME _____ HR _____ P _____
Interval 2: TIME _____ HR _____ P _____
Interval 3: TIME _____ HR _____ P _____
Interval 4: TIME _____ HR _____ P _____
Interval 5: TIME _____ HR _____ P _____

Workout Notes _____

Personal Notes _____

Thursday ■ Date: ___ / ___ / ___

Waking Heart Rate _____

Standing Heart Rate _____

Waking Weight _____ Hours of Sleep _____

Quality of Sleep 1 2 3 4 5 6 7 8 9 10

Mood State 1 2 3 4 5 6 7 8 9 10

Goal _____

Workout _____

Specific Task _____

Actual Workout Time _____

Distance _____ Cadence _____

Average Heart Rate _____ Power _____

Interval 1: TIME _____ HR _____ P _____
Interval 2: TIME _____ HR _____ P _____
Interval 3: TIME _____ HR _____ P _____
Interval 4: TIME _____ HR _____ P _____
Interval 5: TIME _____ HR _____ P _____

Workout Notes _____

Personal Notes _____

Friday ■ Date: ___ / ___ / ___

Waking Heart Rate _____

Standing Heart Rate _____

Waking Weight _____ Hours of Sleep _____

Quality of Sleep 1 2 3 4 5 6 7 8 9 10

Mood State 1 2 3 4 5 6 7 8 9 10

Goal _____

Workout _____

Specific Task _____

Actual Workout Time _____

Distance _____ Cadence _____

Average Heart Rate _____ Power _____

Interval 1: TIME _____ HR _____ P _____
Interval 2: TIME _____ HR _____ P _____
Interval 3: TIME _____ HR _____ P _____
Interval 4: TIME _____ HR _____ P _____
Interval 5: TIME _____ HR _____ P _____

Workout Notes _____

Personal Notes _____

Saturday ■ Date: ___ / ___ / ___

Waking Heart Rate _____

Standing Heart Rate _____

Waking Weight _____ Hours of Sleep _____

Quality of Sleep 1 2 3 4 5 6 7 8 9 10

Mood State 1 2 3 4 5 6 7 8 9 10

Goal _____

Workout _____

Specific Task _____

Actual Workout Time _____

Distance _____ Cadence _____

Average Heart Rate _____ Power _____

Interval 1: TIME _____ HR _____ P _____
Interval 2: TIME _____ HR _____ P _____
Interval 3: TIME _____ HR _____ P _____
Interval 4: TIME _____ HR _____ P _____
Interval 5: TIME _____ HR _____ P _____

Workout Notes _____

Personal Notes _____

Week #

Sunday ■ Date: ___ / ___ / ___

Waking Heart Rate ___

Standing Heart Rate ___

Waking Weight ___ Hours of Sleep ___

Quality of Sleep 1 2 3 4 5 6 7 8 9 10

Mood State 1 2 3 4 5 6 7 8 9 10

Goal ___

Workout ___

Specific Task ___

Actual Workout Time ___

Distance ___ Cadence ___

Average Heart Rate ___ Power ___

Interval 1: TIME ___ HR ___ P ___

Interval 2: TIME ___ HR ___ P ___

Interval 3: TIME ___ HR ___ P ___

Interval 4: TIME ___ HR ___ P ___

Interval 5: TIME ___ HR ___ P ___

Workout Notes ___

Personal Notes ___

Weekly Summary

Hours of Cycling: ___ Year-to-Date: ___

Miles/Kilometers: ___ Year-to-Date: ___

Hours of Strength Training: ___ Year-to-Date: ___

Hours of Other Activities: ___ Year-to-Date: ___

___ Year-to-Date: ___

___ Year-to-Date: ___

___ Year-to-Date: ___

Total Training Hours: ___

Number of Workouts Planned: ___

Number of Workouts Completed: ___

Average Hours of Sleep: ___

Average Quality of Sleep: ___

Average Mood State: ___

Time Spent in Heart Rate/Power Ranges:

CTS RANGES	TIME	CTS RANGES	TIME	OTHER WORKOUTS	TIME
RecoveryMiles™		SteadyState™			
FoundationMiles™		ClimbingRepeats™			
EnduranceMiles™		Max Effort			
Tempo™					

Personal Notes: ___

Weekly Strength Training Record

Exercise	Date:						Date:						Date:					
	SET 1		SET 2		SET 3		SET 1		SET 2		SET 3		SET 1		SET 2		SET 3	
	lbs.	reps	lbs.	reps	lbs.	reps	lbs.	reps	lbs.	reps	lbs.	reps	lbs.	reps	lbs.	reps	lbs.	reps

Race Results

Race #1 _____ Date: __ / __ / __

Time _____ Distance _____

Goal _____

Result _____

Average Heart Rate _____ Power _____

Food/Fluid Intake _____

Personal Notes _____

_____

_____

Race #2 _____ Date: __ / __ / __

Time _____ Distance _____

Goal _____

Result _____

Average Heart Rate _____ Power _____

Food/Fluid Intake _____

Personal Notes _____

_____

_____

Monday ■ Date: ___ / ___ / ___

Waking Heart Rate _____

Standing Heart Rate _____

Waking Weight _____ Hours of Sleep _____

Quality of Sleep   1 2 3 4 5 6 7 8 9 10

Mood State   1 2 3 4 5 6 7 8 9 10

Goal _____

Workout _____

Specific Task _____

Actual Workout Time _____

Distance _____ Cadence _____

Average Heart Rate _____ Power _____

Interval 1: TIME _____ HR _____ P _____

Interval 2: TIME _____ HR _____ P _____

Interval 3: TIME _____ HR _____ P _____

Interval 4: TIME _____ HR _____ P _____

Interval 5: TIME _____ HR _____ P _____

Workout Notes _____

Personal Notes _____

Tuesday ■ Date: ___ / ___ / ___

Waking Heart Rate _____

Standing Heart Rate _____

Waking Weight _____ Hours of Sleep _____

Quality of Sleep   1 2 3 4 5 6 7 8 9 10

Mood State   1 2 3 4 5 6 7 8 9 10

Goal _____

Workout _____

Specific Task _____

Actual Workout Time _____

Distance _____ Cadence _____

Average Heart Rate _____ Power _____

Interval 1: TIME _____ HR _____ P _____

Interval 2: TIME _____ HR _____ P _____

Interval 3: TIME _____ HR _____ P _____

Interval 4: TIME _____ HR _____ P _____

Interval 5: TIME _____ HR _____ P _____

Workout Notes _____

Personal Notes _____

Wednesday ■ Date: ___ / ___ / ___

Waking Heart Rate _____

Standing Heart Rate _____

Waking Weight _____ Hours of Sleep _____

Quality of Sleep   1 2 3 4 5 6 7 8 9 10

Mood State   1 2 3 4 5 6 7 8 9 10

Goal _____

Workout _____

Specific Task _____

Actual Workout Time _____

Distance _____ Cadence _____

Average Heart Rate _____ Power _____

Interval 1: TIME _____ HR _____ P _____

Interval 2: TIME _____ HR _____ P _____

Interval 3: TIME _____ HR _____ P _____

Interval 4: TIME _____ HR _____ P _____

Interval 5: TIME _____ HR _____ P _____

Workout Notes _____

Personal Notes _____

Thursday ■ Date: ___ / ___ / ___

Waking Heart Rate _____

Standing Heart Rate _____

Waking Weight _____ Hours of Sleep _____

Quality of Sleep 1 2 3 4 5 6 7 8 9 10

Mood State 1 2 3 4 5 6 7 8 9 10

Goal _____

Workout _____

Specific Task _____

Actual Workout Time _____

Distance _____ Cadence _____

Average Heart Rate _____ Power _____

Interval 1: TIME _____ HR _____ P _____
Interval 2: TIME _____ HR _____ P _____
Interval 3: TIME _____ HR _____ P _____
Interval 4: TIME _____ HR _____ P _____
Interval 5: TIME _____ HR _____ P _____

Workout Notes _____

Personal Notes _____

Friday ■ Date: ___ / ___ / ___

Waking Heart Rate _____

Standing Heart Rate _____

Waking Weight _____ Hours of Sleep _____

Quality of Sleep 1 2 3 4 5 6 7 8 9 10

Mood State 1 2 3 4 5 6 7 8 9 10

Goal _____

Workout _____

Specific Task _____

Actual Workout Time _____

Distance _____ Cadence _____

Average Heart Rate _____ Power _____

Interval 1: TIME _____ HR _____ P _____
Interval 2: TIME _____ HR _____ P _____
Interval 3: TIME _____ HR _____ P _____
Interval 4: TIME _____ HR _____ P _____
Interval 5: TIME _____ HR _____ P _____

Workout Notes _____

Personal Notes _____

Saturday ■ Date: ___ / ___ / ___

Waking Heart Rate _____

Standing Heart Rate _____

Waking Weight _____ Hours of Sleep _____

Quality of Sleep 1 2 3 4 5 6 7 8 9 10

Mood State 1 2 3 4 5 6 7 8 9 10

Goal _____

Workout _____

Specific Task _____

Actual Workout Time _____

Distance _____ Cadence _____

Average Heart Rate _____ Power _____

Interval 1: TIME _____ HR _____ P _____
Interval 2: TIME _____ HR _____ P _____
Interval 3: TIME _____ HR _____ P _____
Interval 4: TIME _____ HR _____ P _____
Interval 5: TIME _____ HR _____ P _____

Workout Notes _____

Personal Notes _____

Week #: _____

Sunday ■ Date: _____ / _____ / _____

Waking Heart Rate _____

Standing Heart Rate _____

Waking Weight _____ Hours of Sleep _____

Quality of Sleep 1 2 3 4 5 6 7 8 9 10

Mood State 1 2 3 4 5 6 7 8 9 10

Goal _____

Workout _____

Specific Task _____

Actual Workout Time _____

Distance _____ Cadence _____

Average Heart Rate _____ Power _____

Interval 1: TIME _____ HR _____ P _____

Interval 2: TIME _____ HR _____ P _____

Interval 3: TIME _____ HR _____ P _____

Interval 4: TIME _____ HR _____ P _____

Interval 5: TIME _____ HR _____ P _____

Workout Notes _____

Personal Notes _____

Weekly Summary

Hours of Cycling: _____ Year-to-Date: _____

Miles/Kilometers: _____ Year-to-Date: _____

Hours of Strength Training: _____ Year-to-Date: _____

Hours of Other Activities: _____ Year-to-Date: _____

_____ Year-to-Date: _____

_____ Year-to-Date: _____

_____ Year-to-Date: _____

Total Training Hours: _____

Number of Workouts Planned: _____

Number of Workouts Completed: _____

Average Hours of Sleep: _____

Average Quality of Sleep: _____

Average Mood State: _____

Time Spent in Heart Rate/Power Ranges:

CTS RANGES	TIME	CTS RANGES	TIME	OTHER WORKOUTS	TIME
RecoveryMiles™		SteadyState™			
FoundationMiles™		ClimbingRepeats™			
EnduranceMiles™		Max Effort			
Tempo™					

Personal Notes: _____

Weekly Strength Training Record

Exercise	Date:						Date:						Date:					
	SET 1		SET 2		SET 3		SET 1		SET 2		SET 3		SET 1		SET 2		SET 3	
	lbs.	reps	lbs.	reps	lbs.	reps	lbs.	reps	lbs.	reps	lbs.	reps	lbs.	reps	lbs.	reps	lbs.	reps

Race Results

Race #1 _____ Date: __/__/__

Time _____ Distance _____

Goal _____

Result _____

Average Heart Rate _____ Power _____

Food/Fluid Intake _____

Personal Notes _____

_____

_____

Race #2 _____ Date: __/__/__

Time _____ Distance _____

Goal _____

Result _____

Average Heart Rate _____ Power _____

Food/Fluid Intake _____

Personal Notes _____

_____

_____

Week # _____   Goal: _____

Monday ■ Date: ___ / ___ / ___

Waking Heart Rate _____

Standing Heart Rate _____

Waking Weight _____ Hours of Sleep _____

Quality of Sleep   1 2 3 4 5 6 7 8 9 10

Mood State   1 2 3 4 5 6 7 8 9 10

Goal _____

Workout _____

Specific Task _____

Actual Workout Time _____

Distance _____ Cadence _____ Power _____

Average Heart Rate _____

Interval 1: TIME _____ HR _____ P _____
Interval 2: TIME _____ HR _____ P _____
Interval 3: TIME _____ HR _____ P _____
Interval 4: TIME _____ HR _____ P _____
Interval 5: TIME _____ HR _____ P _____

Workout Notes _____

Personal Notes _____

Tuesday ■ Date: ___ / ___ / ___

Waking Heart Rate _____

Standing Heart Rate _____

Waking Weight _____ Hours of Sleep _____

Quality of Sleep   1 2 3 4 5 6 7 8 9 10

Mood State   1 2 3 4 5 6 7 8 9 10

Goal _____

Workout _____

Specific Task _____

Actual Workout Time _____

Distance _____ Cadence _____ Power _____

Average Heart Rate _____

Interval 1: TIME _____ HR _____ P _____
Interval 2: TIME _____ HR _____ P _____
Interval 3: TIME _____ HR _____ P _____
Interval 4: TIME _____ HR _____ P _____
Interval 5: TIME _____ HR _____ P _____

Workout Notes _____

Personal Notes _____

Wednesday ■ Date: ___ / ___ / ___

Waking Heart Rate _____

Standing Heart Rate _____

Waking Weight _____ Hours of Sleep _____

Quality of Sleep   1 2 3 4 5 6 7 8 9 10

Mood State   1 2 3 4 5 6 7 8 9 10

Goal _____

Workout _____

Specific Task _____

Actual Workout Time _____

Distance _____ Cadence _____ Power _____

Average Heart Rate _____

Interval 1: TIME _____ HR _____ P _____
Interval 2: TIME _____ HR _____ P _____
Interval 3: TIME _____ HR _____ P _____
Interval 4: TIME _____ HR _____ P _____
Interval 5: TIME _____ HR _____ P _____

Workout Notes _____

Personal Notes _____

Thursday ■ Date: ___ / ___ / ___

Waking Heart Rate ___

Standing Heart Rate ___

Waking Weight ___ Hours of Sleep ___

Quality of Sleep 1 2 3 4 5 6 7 8 9 10

Mood State 1 2 3 4 5 6 7 8 9 10

Goal ___

Workout ___

Specific Task ___

Actual Workout Time ___

Distance ___ Cadence ___

Average Heart Rate ___ Power ___

Interval 1: TIME ___ HR ___ P ___

Interval 2: TIME ___ HR ___ P ___

Interval 3: TIME ___ HR ___ P ___

Interval 4: TIME ___ HR ___ P ___

Interval 5: TIME ___ HR ___ P ___

Workout Notes ___

Personal Notes ___

Friday ■ Date: ___ / ___ / ___

Waking Heart Rate ___

Standing Heart Rate ___

Waking Weight ___ Hours of Sleep ___

Quality of Sleep 1 2 3 4 5 6 7 8 9 10

Mood State 1 2 3 4 5 6 7 8 9 10

Goal ___

Workout ___

Specific Task ___

Actual Workout Time ___

Distance ___ Cadence ___

Average Heart Rate ___ Power ___

Interval 1: TIME ___ HR ___ P ___

Interval 2: TIME ___ HR ___ P ___

Interval 3: TIME ___ HR ___ P ___

Interval 4: TIME ___ HR ___ P ___

Interval 5: TIME ___ HR ___ P ___

Workout Notes ___

Personal Notes ___

Saturday ■ Date: ___ / ___ / ___

Waking Heart Rate ___

Standing Heart Rate ___

Waking Weight ___ Hours of Sleep ___

Quality of Sleep 1 2 3 4 5 6 7 8 9 10

Mood State 1 2 3 4 5 6 7 8 9 10

Goal ___

Workout ___

Specific Task ___

Actual Workout Time ___

Distance ___ Cadence ___

Average Heart Rate ___ Power ___

Interval 1: TIME ___ HR ___ P ___

Interval 2: TIME ___ HR ___ P ___

Interval 3: TIME ___ HR ___ P ___

Interval 4: TIME ___ HR ___ P ___

Interval 5: TIME ___ HR ___ P ___

Workout Notes ___

Personal Notes ___

Sunday ■ Date: ___ / ___ / ___

Waking Heart Rate ___

Standing Heart Rate ___

Waking Weight ___ Hours of Sleep ___

Quality of Sleep 1 2 3 4 5 6 7 8 9 10

Mood State 1 2 3 4 5 6 7 8 9 10

Goal ___

Workout ___

Specific Task ___

Actual Workout Time ___

Distance ___ Cadence ___

Average Heart Rate ___ Power ___

Interval 1:	TIME ___	HR ___	P ___
Interval 2:	TIME ___	HR ___	P ___
Interval 3:	TIME ___	HR ___	P ___
Interval 4:	TIME ___	HR ___	P ___
Interval 5:	TIME ___	HR ___	P ___

Workout Notes ___

Personal Notes ___

Weekly Summary

Hours of Cycling: ___ Year-to-Date: ___

Miles/Kilometers: ___ Year-to-Date: ___

Hours of Strength Training: ___ Year-to-Date: ___

Hours of Other Activities: ___ Year-to-Date: ___

___ Year-to-Date: ___

___ Year-to-Date: ___

___ Year-to-Date: ___

Total Training Hours: ___

Number of Workouts Planned: ___

Number of Workouts Completed: ___

Average Hours of Sleep: ___

Average Quality of Sleep: ___

Average Mood State: ___

Time Spent in Heart Rate/Power Ranges:

CTS RANGES	TIME	CTS RANGES	TIME	OTHER WORKOUTS	TIME
RecoveryMiles™	___	SteadyState™	___		___
FoundationMiles™	___	ClimbingRepeats™	___		___
EnduranceMiles™	___	Max Effort	___		
Tempo™	___				

Personal Notes: ___

Weekly Strength Training Record

Exercise	Date:			Date:			Date:		
	SET 1 lbs. / reps	SET 2 lbs. / reps	SET 3 lbs. / reps	SET 1 lbs. / reps	SET 2 lbs. / reps	SET 3 lbs. / reps	SET 1 lbs. / reps	SET 2 lbs. / reps	SET 3 lbs. / reps

Race Results

Race #1 _____ Date: ___/___/___

Time _____ Distance _____

Goal _____

Result _____

Average Heart Rate _____ Power _____

Food/Fluid Intake _____

Personal Notes _____

_____

_____

Race #2 _____ Date: ___/___/___

Time _____ Distance _____

Goal _____

Result _____

Average Heart Rate _____ Power _____

Food/Fluid Intake _____

Personal Notes _____

_____

_____

Week # _____ Goal: _____

Monday ▪ Date: ___ / ___ / ___

Waking Heart Rate _____

Standing Heart Rate _____

Waking Weight _____ Hours of Sleep _____

Quality of Sleep 1 2 3 4 5 6 7 8 9 10

Mood State 1 2 3 4 5 6 7 8 9 10

Goal _____

Workout _____

Specific Task _____

Actual Workout Time _____

Distance _____ Cadence _____

Average Heart Rate _____ Power _____

Interval 1:	TIME	HR	P
Interval 2:	TIME	HR	P
Interval 3:	TIME	HR	P
Interval 4:	TIME	HR	P
Interval 5:	TIME	HR	P

Workout Notes _____

Personal Notes _____

Tuesday ▪ Date: ___ / ___ / ___

Waking Heart Rate _____

Standing Heart Rate _____

Waking Weight _____ Hours of Sleep _____

Quality of Sleep 1 2 3 4 5 6 7 8 9 10

Mood State 1 2 3 4 5 6 7 8 9 10

Goal _____

Workout _____

Specific Task _____

Actual Workout Time _____

Distance _____ Cadence _____

Average Heart Rate _____ Power _____

Interval 1:	TIME	HR	P
Interval 2:	TIME	HR	P
Interval 3:	TIME	HR	P
Interval 4:	TIME	HR	P
Interval 5:	TIME	HR	P

Workout Notes _____

Personal Notes _____

Wednesday ▪ Date: ___ / ___ / ___

Waking Heart Rate _____

Standing Heart Rate _____

Waking Weight _____ Hours of Sleep _____

Quality of Sleep 1 2 3 4 5 6 7 8 9 10

Mood State 1 2 3 4 5 6 7 8 9 10

Goal _____

Workout _____

Specific Task _____

Actual Workout Time _____

Distance _____ Cadence _____

Average Heart Rate _____ Power _____

Interval 1:	TIME	HR	P
Interval 2:	TIME	HR	P
Interval 3:	TIME	HR	P
Interval 4:	TIME	HR	P
Interval 5:	TIME	HR	P

Workout Notes _____

Personal Notes _____

Thursday ■ Date: ___ / ___ / ___

Waking Heart Rate _____

Standing Heart Rate _____

Waking Weight _____ Hours of Sleep _____

Quality of Sleep 1 2 3 4 5 6 7 8 9 10

Mood State 1 2 3 4 5 6 7 8 9 10

Goal _____

Workout _____

Specific Task _____

Actual Workout Time _____

Distance _____ Cadence _____

Average Heart Rate _____ Power _____

Interval 1: TIME _____ HR _____ P _____
Interval 2: TIME _____ HR _____ P _____
Interval 3: TIME _____ HR _____ P _____
Interval 4: TIME _____ HR _____ P _____
Interval 5: TIME _____ HR _____ P _____

Workout Notes _____

Personal Notes _____

Friday ■ Date: ___ / ___ / ___

Waking Heart Rate _____

Standing Heart Rate _____

Waking Weight _____ Hours of Sleep _____

Quality of Sleep 1 2 3 4 5 6 7 8 9 10

Mood State 1 2 3 4 5 6 7 8 9 10

Goal _____

Workout _____

Specific Task _____

Actual Workout Time _____

Distance _____ Cadence _____

Average Heart Rate _____ Power _____

Interval 1: TIME _____ HR _____ P _____
Interval 2: TIME _____ HR _____ P _____
Interval 3: TIME _____ HR _____ P _____
Interval 4: TIME _____ HR _____ P _____
Interval 5: TIME _____ HR _____ P _____

Workout Notes _____

Personal Notes _____

Saturday ■ Date: ___ / ___ / ___

Waking Heart Rate _____

Standing Heart Rate _____

Waking Weight _____ Hours of Sleep _____

Quality of Sleep 1 2 3 4 5 6 7 8 9 10

Mood State 1 2 3 4 5 6 7 8 9 10

Goal _____

Workout _____

Specific Task _____

Actual Workout Time _____

Distance _____ Cadence _____

Average Heart Rate _____ Power _____

Interval 1: TIME _____ HR _____ P _____
Interval 2: TIME _____ HR _____ P _____
Interval 3: TIME _____ HR _____ P _____
Interval 4: TIME _____ HR _____ P _____
Interval 5: TIME _____ HR _____ P _____

Workout Notes _____

Personal Notes _____

Sunday ■ Date: ___ / ___ / ___

Waking Heart Rate ___

Standing Heart Rate ___

Waking Weight ___ Hours of Sleep ___

Quality of Sleep 1 2 3 4 5 6 7 8 9 10

Mood State 1 2 3 4 5 6 7 8 9 10

Goal ___

Workout ___

Specific Task ___

Actual Workout Time ___

Distance ___ Cadence ___

Average Heart Rate ___ Power ___

Interval 1: TIME ___ HR ___ P ___

Interval 2: TIME ___ HR ___ P ___

Interval 3: TIME ___ HR ___ P ___

Interval 4: TIME ___ HR ___ P ___

Interval 5: TIME ___ HR ___ P ___

Workout Notes ___

Personal Notes ___

Weekly Summary

Hours of Cycling: ___ Year-to-Date: ___

Miles/Kilometers: ___ Year-to-Date: ___

Hours of Strength Training: ___ Year-to-Date: ___

Hours of Other Activities: ___

___ Year-to-Date: ___

___ Year-to-Date: ___

___ Year-to-Date: ___

___ Year-to-Date: ___

Total Training Hours: ___

Number of Workouts Planned: ___

Number of Workouts Completed: ___

Average Hours of Sleep: ___

Average Quality of Sleep: ___

Average Mood State: ___

Time Spent in Heart Rate/Power Ranges:

CTS RANGES	TIME	CTS RANGES	TIME	OTHER WORKOUTS	TIME
RecoveryMiles™		SteadyState™			
FoundationMiles™		ClimbingRepeats™			
EnduranceMiles™		Max Effort			
Tempo™					

Personal Notes: ___

Weekly Strength Training Record

Exercise	Date:						Date:						Date:					
	SET 1		SET 2		SET 3		SET 1		SET 2		SET 3		SET 1		SET 2		SET 3	
	lbs. / reps		lbs. / reps		lbs. / reps		lbs. / reps		lbs. / reps		lbs. / reps		lbs. / reps		lbs. / reps		lbs. / reps	

Race Results

Race #1 _____ Date: ___ / ___ / ___

Time _____ Distance _____

Goal _____

Result _____

Average Heart Rate _____ Power _____

Food/Fluid Intake _____

Personal Notes _____

_____

_____

Race #2 _____ Date: ___ / ___ / ___

Time _____ Distance _____

Goal _____

Result _____

Average Heart Rate _____ Power _____

Food/Fluid Intake _____

Personal Notes _____

_____

_____

Monday ■ Date: ___ / ___ / ___

Waking Heart Rate _____

Standing Heart Rate _____

Waking Weight _____ Hours of Sleep _____

Quality of Sleep   1 2 3 4 5 6 7 8 9 10

Mood State   1 2 3 4 5 6 7 8 9 10

Goal _____

Workout _____

Specific Task _____

Actual Workout Time _____

Distance _____ Cadence _____ Power _____

Average Heart Rate _____

Interval 1:	TIME ____	HR ____	P. ____
Interval 2:	TIME ____	HR ____	P. ____
Interval 3:	TIME ____	HR ____	P. ____
Interval 4:	TIME ____	HR ____	P. ____
Interval 5:	TIME ____	HR ____	P. ____

Workout Notes _____

Personal Notes _____

Tuesday ■ Date: ___ / ___ / ___

Waking Heart Rate _____

Standing Heart Rate _____

Waking Weight _____ Hours of Sleep _____

Quality of Sleep   1 2 3 4 5 6 7 8 9 10

Mood State   1 2 3 4 5 6 7 8 9 10

Goal _____

Workout _____

Specific Task _____

Actual Workout Time _____

Distance _____ Cadence _____ Power _____

Average Heart Rate _____

Interval 1:	TIME ____	HR ____	P. ____
Interval 2:	TIME ____	HR ____	P. ____
Interval 3:	TIME ____	HR ____	P. ____
Interval 4:	TIME ____	HR ____	P. ____
Interval 5:	TIME ____	HR ____	P. ____

Workout Notes _____

Personal Notes _____

Wednesday ■ Date: ___ / ___ / ___

Waking Heart Rate _____

Standing Heart Rate _____

Waking Weight _____ Hours of Sleep _____

Quality of Sleep   1 2 3 4 5 6 7 8 9 10

Mood State   1 2 3 4 5 6 7 8 9 10

Goal _____

Workout _____

Specific Task _____

Actual Workout Time _____

Distance _____ Cadence _____ Power _____

Average Heart Rate _____

Interval 1:	TIME ____	HR ____	P. ____
Interval 2:	TIME ____	HR ____	P. ____
Interval 3:	TIME ____	HR ____	P. ____
Interval 4:	TIME ____	HR ____	P. ____
Interval 5:	TIME ____	HR ____	P. ____

Workout Notes _____

Personal Notes _____

Week #

Thursday ■ Date: ___ / ___ / ___

Waking Heart Rate _____

Standing Heart Rate _____

Waking Weight _____ Hours of Sleep _____

Quality of Sleep 1 2 3 4 5 6 7 8 9 10

Mood State 1 2 3 4 5 6 7 8 9 10

Goal _____

Workout _____

Specific Task _____

Actual Workout Time _____

Distance _____ Cadence _____ Power _____

Average Heart Rate _____

Interval 1:	TIME _____	HR _____	P _____
Interval 2:	TIME _____	HR _____	P _____
Interval 3:	TIME _____	HR _____	P _____
Interval 4:	TIME _____	HR _____	P _____
Interval 5:	TIME _____	HR _____	P _____

Workout Notes _____

Personal Notes _____

Friday ■ Date: ___ / ___ / ___

Waking Heart Rate _____

Standing Heart Rate _____

Waking Weight _____ Hours of Sleep _____

Quality of Sleep 1 2 3 4 5 6 7 8 9 10

Mood State 1 2 3 4 5 6 7 8 9 10

Goal _____

Workout _____

Specific Task _____

Actual Workout Time _____

Distance _____ Cadence _____ Power _____

Average Heart Rate _____

Interval 1:	TIME _____	HR _____	P _____
Interval 2:	TIME _____	HR _____	P _____
Interval 3:	TIME _____	HR _____	P _____
Interval 4:	TIME _____	HR _____	P _____
Interval 5:	TIME _____	HR _____	P _____

Workout Notes _____

Personal Notes _____

Saturday ■ Date: ___ / ___ / ___

Waking Heart Rate _____

Standing Heart Rate _____

Waking Weight _____ Hours of Sleep _____

Quality of Sleep 1 2 3 4 5 6 7 8 9 10

Mood State 1 2 3 4 5 6 7 8 9 10

Goal _____

Workout _____

Specific Task _____

Actual Workout Time _____

Distance _____ Cadence _____ Power _____

Average Heart Rate _____

Interval 1:	TIME _____	HR _____	P _____
Interval 2:	TIME _____	HR _____	P _____
Interval 3:	TIME _____	HR _____	P _____
Interval 4:	TIME _____	HR _____	P _____
Interval 5:	TIME _____	HR _____	P _____

Workout Notes _____

Personal Notes _____

Sunday ■ Date: ___ / ___ / ___

Waking Heart Rate _____

Standing Heart Rate _____

Waking Weight _____ Hours of Sleep _____

Quality of Sleep 1 2 3 4 5 6 7 8 9 10

Mood State 1 2 3 4 5 6 7 8 9 10

Goal _____

Workout _____

Specific Task _____

Actual Workout Time _____

Distance _____ Cadence _____

Average Heart Rate _____ Power _____

Interval 1:	TIME ____	HR ____	P ____
Interval 2:	TIME ____	HR ____	P ____
Interval 3:	TIME ____	HR ____	P ____
Interval 4:	TIME ____	HR ____	P ____
Interval 5:	TIME ____	HR ____	P ____

Workout Notes _____

Personal Notes _____

Weekly Summary

Hours of Cycling: _____ Year-to-Date: _____

Miles/Kilometers: _____ Year-to-Date: _____

Hours of Strength Training: _____ Year-to-Date: _____

Hours of Other Activities: _____ Year-to-Date: _____

_____ Year-to-Date: _____

_____ Year-to-Date: _____

_____ Year-to-Date: _____

_____ Year-to-Date: _____

Total Training Hours: _____

Number of Workouts Planned: _____

Number of Workouts Completed: _____

Average Hours of Sleep: _____

Average Quality of Sleep: _____

Average Mood State: _____

Time Spent in Heart Rate/Power Ranges:

CTS RANGES	TIME	CTS RANGES	TIME	OTHER WORKOUTS	TIME
RecoveryMiles™	____	SteadyState™	____		____
FoundationMiles™	____	ClimbingRepeats™	____		____
EnduranceMiles™	____	Max Effort	____		____
Tempo™	____				

Personal Notes: _____

Weekly Strength Training Record

Exercise	Date:						Date:						Date:					
	SET 1		SET 2		SET 3		SET 1		SET 2		SET 3		SET 1		SET 2		SET 3	
	lbs.	reps	lbs.	reps	lbs.	reps	lbs.	reps	lbs.	reps	lbs.	reps	lbs.	reps	lbs.	reps	lbs.	reps

Race Results

Race #1 _____ Date: ___ / ___ / ___

Time _____ Distance _____

Goal _____

Result _____

Average Heart Rate _____ Power _____

Food/Fluid Intake _____

Personal Notes _____

_____

_____

Race #2 _____ Date: ___ / ___ / ___

Time _____ Distance _____

Goal _____

Result _____

Average Heart Rate _____ Power _____

Food/Fluid Intake _____

Personal Notes _____

_____

_____

Week # _____ Goal: _____

Monday ■ Date: ___ / ___ / ___

Waking Heart Rate _____
Standing Heart Rate _____
Waking Weight _____ Hours of Sleep _____
Quality of Sleep 1 2 3 4 5 6 7 8 9 10

Mood State 1 2 3 4 5 6 7 8 9 10

Goal _____
Workout _____
Specific Task _____
Actual Workout Time _____
Distance _____ Cadence _____
Average Heart Rate _____ Power _____

Interval 1: TIME _____ HR _____ P _____
Interval 2: TIME _____ HR _____ P _____
Interval 3: TIME _____ HR _____ P _____
Interval 4: TIME _____ HR _____ P _____
Interval 5: TIME _____ HR _____ P _____

Workout Notes _____

Personal Notes _____

Tuesday ■ Date: ___ / ___ / ___

Waking Heart Rate _____
Standing Heart Rate _____
Waking Weight _____ Hours of Sleep _____
Quality of Sleep 1 2 3 4 5 6 7 8 9 10

Mood State 1 2 3 4 5 6 7 8 9 10

Goal _____
Workout _____
Specific Task _____
Actual Workout Time _____
Distance _____ Cadence _____
Average Heart Rate _____ Power _____

Interval 1: TIME _____ HR _____ P _____
Interval 2: TIME _____ HR _____ P _____
Interval 3: TIME _____ HR _____ P _____
Interval 4: TIME _____ HR _____ P _____
Interval 5: TIME _____ HR _____ P _____

Workout Notes _____

Personal Notes _____

Wednesday ■ Date: ___ / ___ / ___

Waking Heart Rate _____
Standing Heart Rate _____
Waking Weight _____ Hours of Sleep _____
Quality of Sleep 1 2 3 4 5 6 7 8 9 10

Mood State 1 2 3 4 5 6 7 8 9 10

Goal _____
Workout _____
Specific Task _____
Actual Workout Time _____
Distance _____ Cadence _____
Average Heart Rate _____ Power _____

Interval 1: TIME _____ HR _____ P _____
Interval 2: TIME _____ HR _____ P _____
Interval 3: TIME _____ HR _____ P _____
Interval 4: TIME _____ HR _____ P _____
Interval 5: TIME _____ HR _____ P _____

Workout Notes _____

Personal Notes _____

Week #

Thursday ■ Date: ___ / ___ / ___

Waking Heart Rate ___
Standing Heart Rate ___
Waking Weight ___ Hours of Sleep ___
Quality of Sleep 1 2 3 4 5 6 7 8 9 10

Mood State 1 2 3 4 5 6 7 8 9 10

Goal ___
Workout ___
Specific Task ___
Actual Workout Time ___
Distance ___ Cadence ___
Average Heart Rate ___ Power ___

Interval 1: TIME ___ HR ___ P ___
Interval 2: TIME ___ HR ___ P ___
Interval 3: TIME ___ HR ___ P ___
Interval 4: TIME ___ HR ___ P ___
Interval 5: TIME ___ HR ___ P ___

Workout Notes ___

Personal Notes ___

Friday ■ Date: ___ / ___ / ___

Waking Heart Rate ___
Standing Heart Rate ___
Waking Weight ___ Hours of Sleep ___
Quality of Sleep 1 2 3 4 5 6 7 8 9 10

Mood State 1 2 3 4 5 6 7 8 9 10

Goal ___
Workout ___
Specific Task ___
Actual Workout Time ___
Distance ___ Cadence ___
Average Heart Rate ___ Power ___

Interval 1: TIME ___ HR ___ P ___
Interval 2: TIME ___ HR ___ P ___
Interval 3: TIME ___ HR ___ P ___
Interval 4: TIME ___ HR ___ P ___
Interval 5: TIME ___ HR ___ P ___

Workout Notes ___

Personal Notes ___

Saturday ■ Date: ___ / ___ / ___

Waking Heart Rate ___
Standing Heart Rate ___
Waking Weight ___ Hours of Sleep ___
Quality of Sleep 1 2 3 4 5 6 7 8 9 10

Mood State 1 2 3 4 5 6 7 8 9 10

Goal ___
Workout ___
Specific Task ___
Actual Workout Time ___
Distance ___ Cadence ___
Average Heart Rate ___ Power ___

Interval 1: TIME ___ HR ___ P ___
Interval 2: TIME ___ HR ___ P ___
Interval 3: TIME ___ HR ___ P ___
Interval 4: TIME ___ HR ___ P ___
Interval 5: TIME ___ HR ___ P ___

Workout Notes ___

Personal Notes ___

Week # _____

Sunday ■ Date: ___ / ___ / ___

Waking Heart Rate _____

Standing Heart Rate _____

Waking Weight _____ Hours of Sleep _____

Quality of Sleep 1 2 3 4 5 6 7 8 9 10

Mood State 1 2 3 4 5 6 7 8 9 10

Goal _____

Workout _____

Specific Task _____

Actual Workout Time _____

Distance _____ Cadence _____

Average Heart Rate _____ Power _____

Interval 1: TIME _____ HR _____ P _____
Interval 2: TIME _____ HR _____ P _____
Interval 3: TIME _____ HR _____ P _____
Interval 4: TIME _____ HR _____ P _____
Interval 5: TIME _____ HR _____ P _____

Workout Notes _____

Personal Notes _____

Weekly Summary

Hours of Cycling: _____ Year-to-Date: _____

Miles/Kilometers: _____ Year-to-Date: _____

Hours of Strength Training: _____ Year-to-Date: _____

Hours of Other Activities: _____ Year-to-Date: _____

_____ Year-to-Date: _____

Total Training Hours: _____ Year-to-Date: _____

Number of Workouts Planned: _____

Number of Workouts Completed: _____

Average Hours of Sleep: _____

Average Quality of Sleep: _____

Average Mood State: _____

Time Spent in Heart Rate/Power Ranges:

CTS RANGES	TIME	CTS RANGES	TIME	OTHER WORKOUTS	TIME
RecoveryMiles™		SteadyState™			
FoundationMiles™		ClimbingRepeats™			
EnduranceMiles™		Max Effort			
Tempo™					

Personal Notes: _____

Weekly Strength Training Record

Exercise	Date:						Date:						Date:					
	SET 1		SET 2		SET 3		SET 1		SET 2		SET 3		SET 1		SET 2		SET 3	
	lbs.	reps	lbs.	reps	lbs.	reps	lbs.	reps	lbs.	reps	lbs.	reps	lbs.	reps	lbs.	reps	lbs.	reps

Race Results

Race #1 _____ Date: ___ / ___ / ___

Time _____ Distance _____

Goal _____

Result _____

Average Heart Rate _____ Power _____

Food/Fluid Intake _____

Personal Notes _____

_____

_____

Race #2 _____ Date: ___ / ___ / ___

Time _____ Distance _____

Goal _____

Result _____

Average Heart Rate _____ Power _____

Food/Fluid Intake _____

Personal Notes _____

_____

_____

Week # _____ Goal: _____

Monday ■ Date: ___ / ___ / ___

Waking Heart Rate _____
Standing Heart Rate _____
Waking Weight _____ Hours of Sleep _____
Quality of Sleep 1 2 3 4 5 6 7 8 9 10

Mood State 1 2 3 4 5 6 7 8 9 10

Goal _____
Workout _____
Specific Task _____
Actual Workout Time _____
Distance _____ Cadence _____
Average Heart Rate _____ Power _____

Interval 1: TIME ____ HR ____ P ____
Interval 2: TIME ____ HR ____ P ____
Interval 3: TIME ____ HR ____ P ____
Interval 4: TIME ____ HR ____ P ____
Interval 5: TIME ____ HR ____ P ____
Workout Notes _____

Personal Notes _____

Tuesday ■ Date: ___ / ___ / ___

Waking Heart Rate _____
Standing Heart Rate _____
Waking Weight _____ Hours of Sleep _____
Quality of Sleep 1 2 3 4 5 6 7 8 9 10

Mood State 1 2 3 4 5 6 7 8 9 10

Goal _____
Workout _____
Specific Task _____
Actual Workout Time _____
Distance _____ Cadence _____
Average Heart Rate _____ Power _____

Interval 1: TIME ____ HR ____ P ____
Interval 2: TIME ____ HR ____ P ____
Interval 3: TIME ____ HR ____ P ____
Interval 4: TIME ____ HR ____ P ____
Interval 5: TIME ____ HR ____ P ____
Workout Notes _____

Personal Notes _____

Wednesday ■ Date: ___ / ___ / ___

Waking Heart Rate _____
Standing Heart Rate _____
Waking Weight _____ Hours of Sleep _____
Quality of Sleep 1 2 3 4 5 6 7 8 9 10

Mood State 1 2 3 4 5 6 7 8 9 10

Goal _____
Workout _____
Specific Task _____
Actual Workout Time _____
Distance _____ Cadence _____
Average Heart Rate _____ Power _____

Interval 1: TIME ____ HR ____ P ____
Interval 2: TIME ____ HR ____ P ____
Interval 3: TIME ____ HR ____ P ____
Interval 4: TIME ____ HR ____ P ____
Interval 5: TIME ____ HR ____ P ____
Workout Notes _____

Personal Notes _____

Thursday ■ Date: ___ / ___ / ___

Waking Heart Rate _____

Standing Heart Rate _____

Waking Weight _____ Hours of Sleep _____

Quality of Sleep 1 2 3 4 5 6 7 8 9 10

Mood State 1 2 3 4 5 6 7 8 9 10

Goal _____

Workout _____

Specific Task _____

Actual Workout Time _____

Distance _____ Cadence _____

Average Heart Rate _____ Power _____

Interval 1: TIME _____ HR _____ P _____
Interval 2: TIME _____ HR _____ P _____
Interval 3: TIME _____ HR _____ P _____
Interval 4: TIME _____ HR _____ P _____
Interval 5: TIME _____ HR _____ P _____

Workout Notes _____

Personal Notes _____

Friday ■ Date: ___ / ___ / ___

Waking Heart Rate _____

Standing Heart Rate _____

Waking Weight _____ Hours of Sleep _____

Quality of Sleep 1 2 3 4 5 6 7 8 9 10

Mood State 1 2 3 4 5 6 7 8 9 10

Goal _____

Workout _____

Specific Task _____

Actual Workout Time _____

Distance _____ Cadence _____

Average Heart Rate _____ Power _____

Interval 1: TIME _____ HR _____ P _____
Interval 2: TIME _____ HR _____ P _____
Interval 3: TIME _____ HR _____ P _____
Interval 4: TIME _____ HR _____ P _____
Interval 5: TIME _____ HR _____ P _____

Workout Notes _____

Personal Notes _____

Saturday ■ Date: ___ / ___ / ___

Waking Heart Rate _____

Standing Heart Rate _____

Waking Weight _____ Hours of Sleep _____

Quality of Sleep 1 2 3 4 5 6 7 8 9 10

Mood State 1 2 3 4 5 6 7 8 9 10

Goal _____

Workout _____

Specific Task _____

Actual Workout Time _____

Distance _____ Cadence _____

Average Heart Rate _____ Power _____

Interval 1: TIME _____ HR _____ P _____
Interval 2: TIME _____ HR _____ P _____
Interval 3: TIME _____ HR _____ P _____
Interval 4: TIME _____ HR _____ P _____
Interval 5: TIME _____ HR _____ P _____

Workout Notes _____

Personal Notes _____

Sunday ■ Date: ___ / ___ / ___

Waking Heart Rate _____

Standing Heart Rate _____

Waking Weight _____ Hours of Sleep _____

Quality of Sleep 1 2 3 4 5 6 7 8 9 10

Mood State 1 2 3 4 5 6 7 8 9 10

_____

Goal _____

Workout _____

Specific Task _____

Actual Workout Time _____

Distance _____ Cadence _____

Average Heart Rate _____ Power _____

Interval 1: TIME _____ HR _____ P _____

Interval 2: TIME _____ HR _____ P _____

Interval 3: TIME _____ HR _____ P _____

Interval 4: TIME _____ HR _____ P _____

Interval 5: TIME _____ HR _____ P _____

Workout Notes _____

_____

Personal Notes _____

_____

Weekly Summary

Hours of Cycling: _____ Year-to-Date: _____

Miles/Kilometers: _____ Year-to-Date: _____

Hours of Strength Training: _____ Year-to-Date: _____

Hours of Other Activities: _____ Year-to-Date: _____

_____ Year-to-Date: _____

_____ Year-to-Date: _____

_____ Year-to-Date: _____

Total Training Hours: _____

Number of Workouts Planned: _____

Number of Workouts Completed: _____

Average Hours of Sleep: _____

Average Quality of Sleep: _____

Average Mood State: _____

Time Spent in Heart Rate/Power Ranges:

CTS RANGES	TIME	CTS RANGES	TIME	OTHER WORKOUTS	TIME
RecoveryMiles™		SteadyState™			
FoundationMiles™		ClimbingRepeats™			
EnduranceMiles™		Max Effort			
Tempo™					

Personal Notes: _____

_____

Weekly Strength Training Record

Exercise	Date:						Date:						Date:					
	SET 1		SET 2		SET 3		SET 1		SET 2		SET 3		SET 1		SET 2		SET 3	
	lbs.	reps	lbs.	reps	lbs.	reps	lbs.	reps	lbs.	reps	lbs.	reps	lbs.	reps	lbs.	reps	lbs.	reps

Race Results

Race #1 _____ Date: ___ / ___ / ___

Time _____ Distance _____

Goal _____

Result _____

Average Heart Rate _____ Power _____

Food/Fluid Intake _____

Personal Notes _____

_____

_____

Race #2 _____ Date: ___ / ___ / ___

Time _____ Distance _____

Goal _____

Result _____

Average Heart Rate _____ Power _____

Food/Fluid Intake _____

Personal Notes _____

_____

_____

Week # _____ Goal: _____

Monday ▪ Date: ___ / ___ / ___

Waking Heart Rate _____
Standing Heart Rate _____
Waking Weight _____ Hours of Sleep _____
Quality of Sleep 1 2 3 4 5 6 7 8 9 10

Mood State 1 2 3 4 5 6 7 8 9 10

Goal _____
Workout _____
Specific Task _____
Actual Workout Time _____
Distance _____ Cadence _____
Average Heart Rate _____ Power _____

Interval 1: TIME _____ HR _____ P _____
Interval 2: TIME _____ HR _____ P _____
Interval 3: TIME _____ HR _____ P _____
Interval 4: TIME _____ HR _____ P _____
Interval 5: TIME _____ HR _____ P _____

Workout Notes _____

Personal Notes _____

Tuesday ▪ Date: ___ / ___ / ___

Waking Heart Rate _____
Standing Heart Rate _____
Waking Weight _____ Hours of Sleep _____
Quality of Sleep 1 2 3 4 5 6 7 8 9 10

Mood State 1 2 3 4 5 6 7 8 9 10

Goal _____
Workout _____
Specific Task _____
Actual Workout Time _____
Distance _____ Cadence _____
Average Heart Rate _____ Power _____

Interval 1: TIME _____ HR _____ P _____
Interval 2: TIME _____ HR _____ P _____
Interval 3: TIME _____ HR _____ P _____
Interval 4: TIME _____ HR _____ P _____
Interval 5: TIME _____ HR _____ P _____

Workout Notes _____

Personal Notes _____

Wednesday ▪ Date: ___ / ___ / ___

Waking Heart Rate _____
Standing Heart Rate _____
Waking Weight _____ Hours of Sleep _____
Quality of Sleep 1 2 3 4 5 6 7 8 9 10

Mood State 1 2 3 4 5 6 7 8 9 10

Goal _____
Workout _____
Specific Task _____
Actual Workout Time _____
Distance _____ Cadence _____
Average Heart Rate _____ Power _____

Interval 1: TIME _____ HR _____ P _____
Interval 2: TIME _____ HR _____ P _____
Interval 3: TIME _____ HR _____ P _____
Interval 4: TIME _____ HR _____ P _____
Interval 5: TIME _____ HR _____ P _____

Workout Notes _____

Personal Notes _____

Thursday ■ Date: ___ / ___ / ___

Waking Heart Rate _____

Standing Heart Rate _____

Waking Weight _____ Hours of Sleep _____

Quality of Sleep 1 2 3 4 5 6 7 8 9 10

Mood State 1 2 3 4 5 6 7 8 9 10

Goal _____

Workout _____

Specific Task _____

Actual Workout Time _____

Distance _____ Cadence _____

Average Heart Rate _____ Power _____

Interval 1: TIME _____ HR _____ P _____
Interval 2: TIME _____ HR _____ P _____
Interval 3: TIME _____ HR _____ P _____
Interval 4: TIME _____ HR _____ P _____
Interval 5: TIME _____ HR _____ P _____

Workout Notes _____

Personal Notes _____

Friday ■ Date: ___ / ___ / ___

Waking Heart Rate _____

Standing Heart Rate _____

Waking Weight _____ Hours of Sleep _____

Quality of Sleep 1 2 3 4 5 6 7 8 9 10

Mood State 1 2 3 4 5 6 7 8 9 10

Goal _____

Workout _____

Specific Task _____

Actual Workout Time _____

Distance _____ Cadence _____

Average Heart Rate _____ Power _____

Interval 1: TIME _____ HR _____ P _____
Interval 2: TIME _____ HR _____ P _____
Interval 3: TIME _____ HR _____ P _____
Interval 4: TIME _____ HR _____ P _____
Interval 5: TIME _____ HR _____ P _____

Workout Notes _____

Personal Notes _____

Saturday ■ Date: ___ / ___ / ___

Waking Heart Rate _____

Standing Heart Rate _____

Waking Weight _____ Hours of Sleep _____

Quality of Sleep 1 2 3 4 5 6 7 8 9 10

Mood State 1 2 3 4 5 6 7 8 9 10

Goal _____

Workout _____

Specific Task _____

Actual Workout Time _____

Distance _____ Cadence _____

Average Heart Rate _____ Power _____

Interval 1: TIME _____ HR _____ P _____
Interval 2: TIME _____ HR _____ P _____
Interval 3: TIME _____ HR _____ P _____
Interval 4: TIME _____ HR _____ P _____
Interval 5: TIME _____ HR _____ P _____

Workout Notes _____

Personal Notes _____

Sunday ■ Date: ___ / ___ / ___

Waking Heart Rate _____

Standing Heart Rate _____

Waking Weight _____ Hours of Sleep _____

Quality of Sleep   1 2 3 4 5 6 7 8 9 10

Mood State   1 2 3 4 5 6 7 8 9 10

Goal _____

Workout _____

Specific Task _____

Actual Workout Time _____

Distance _____ Cadence _____

Average Heart Rate _____ Power _____

Interval 1:   TIME _____   HR _____   P _____

Interval 2:   TIME _____   HR _____   P _____

Interval 3:   TIME _____   HR _____   P _____

Interval 4:   TIME _____   HR _____   P _____

Interval 5:   TIME _____   HR _____   P _____

Workout Notes _____

Personal Notes _____

Weekly Summary

Hours of Cycling: _____   Year-to-Date: _____

Miles/Kilometers: _____   Year-to-Date: _____

Hours of Strength Training: _____   Year-to-Date: _____

Hours of Other Activities: _____

_____   Year-to-Date: _____

_____   Year-to-Date: _____

_____   Year-to-Date: _____

_____   Year-to-Date: _____

Total Training Hours: _____

Number of Workouts Planned: _____

Number of Workouts Completed: _____

Average Hours of Sleep: _____

Average Quality of Sleep: _____

Average Mood State: _____

Time Spent in Heart Rate/Power Ranges:

CTS RANGES	TIME	CTS RANGES	TIME	OTHER WORKOUTS	TIME
RecoveryMiles™		SteadyState™			
FoundationMiles™		ClimbingRepeats™			
EnduranceMiles™		Max Effort			
Tempo™					

Personal Notes: _____

Week # _____

Weekly Strength Training Record

Exercise	Date:						Date:						Date:					
	SET 1		SET 2		SET 3		SET 1		SET 2		SET 3		SET 1		SET 2		SET 3	
	lbs.	reps	lbs.	reps	lbs.	reps	lbs.	reps	lbs.	reps	lbs.	reps	lbs.	reps	lbs.	reps	lbs.	reps

Race Results

Race #1 _____ Date: ___ / ___ / ___

Time _____ Distance _____

Goal _____

Result _____

Average Heart Rate _____ Power _____

Food/Fluid Intake _____

Personal Notes _____

_____

_____

Race #2 _____ Date: ___ / ___ / ___

Time _____ Distance _____

Goal _____

Result _____

Average Heart Rate _____ Power _____

Food/Fluid Intake _____

Personal Notes _____

_____

_____

Week # _____   Goal: _____

Monday ■ Date: ___ / ___ / ___

Waking Heart Rate _____
Standing Heart Rate _____
Waking Weight _____ Hours of Sleep _____
Quality of Sleep 1 2 3 4 5 6 7 8 9 10

Mood State 1 2 3 4 5 6 7 8 9 10

Goal _____
Workout _____
Specific Task _____
Actual Workout Time _____
Distance _____ Cadence _____
Average Heart Rate _____ Power _____

Interval 1: TIME _____ HR _____ P _____
Interval 2: TIME _____ HR _____ P _____
Interval 3: TIME _____ HR _____ P _____
Interval 4: TIME _____ HR _____ P _____
Interval 5: TIME _____ HR _____ P _____
Workout Notes _____

Personal Notes _____

Tuesday ■ Date: ___ / ___ / ___

Waking Heart Rate _____
Standing Heart Rate _____
Waking Weight _____ Hours of Sleep _____
Quality of Sleep 1 2 3 4 5 6 7 8 9 10

Mood State 1 2 3 4 5 6 7 8 9 10

Goal _____
Workout _____
Specific Task _____
Actual Workout Time _____
Distance _____ Cadence _____
Average Heart Rate _____ Power _____

Interval 1: TIME _____ HR _____ P _____
Interval 2: TIME _____ HR _____ P _____
Interval 3: TIME _____ HR _____ P _____
Interval 4: TIME _____ HR _____ P _____
Interval 5: TIME _____ HR _____ P _____
Workout Notes _____

Personal Notes _____

Wednesday ■ Date: ___ / ___ / ___

Waking Heart Rate _____
Standing Heart Rate _____
Waking Weight _____ Hours of Sleep _____
Quality of Sleep 1 2 3 4 5 6 7 8 9 10

Mood State 1 2 3 4 5 6 7 8 9 10

Goal _____
Workout _____
Specific Task _____
Actual Workout Time _____
Distance _____ Cadence _____
Average Heart Rate _____ Power _____

Interval 1: TIME _____ HR _____ P _____
Interval 2: TIME _____ HR _____ P _____
Interval 3: TIME _____ HR _____ P _____
Interval 4: TIME _____ HR _____ P _____
Interval 5: TIME _____ HR _____ P _____
Workout Notes _____

Personal Notes _____

Week #

Thursday ■ Date: ___ / ___ / ___

Waking Heart Rate _____

Standing Heart Rate _____

Waking Weight _____ Hours of Sleep _____

Quality of Sleep 1 2 3 4 5 6 7 8 9 10

Mood State 1 2 3 4 5 6 7 8 9 10

Goal _____

Workout _____

Specific Task _____

Actual Workout Time _____

Distance _____ Cadence _____

Average Heart Rate _____ Power _____

Interval 1: TIME _____ HR _____ P _____
Interval 2: TIME _____ HR _____ P _____
Interval 3: TIME _____ HR _____ P _____
Interval 4: TIME _____ HR _____ P _____
Interval 5: TIME _____ HR _____ P _____

Workout Notes _____

Personal Notes _____

Friday ■ Date: ___ / ___ / ___

Waking Heart Rate _____

Standing Heart Rate _____

Waking Weight _____ Hours of Sleep _____

Quality of Sleep 1 2 3 4 5 6 7 8 9 10

Mood State 1 2 3 4 5 6 7 8 9 10

Goal _____

Workout _____

Specific Task _____

Actual Workout Time _____

Distance _____ Cadence _____

Average Heart Rate _____ Power _____

Interval 1: TIME _____ HR _____ P _____
Interval 2: TIME _____ HR _____ P _____
Interval 3: TIME _____ HR _____ P _____
Interval 4: TIME _____ HR _____ P _____
Interval 5: TIME _____ HR _____ P _____

Workout Notes _____

Personal Notes _____

Saturday ■ Date: ___ / ___ / ___

Waking Heart Rate _____

Standing Heart Rate _____

Waking Weight _____ Hours of Sleep _____

Quality of Sleep 1 2 3 4 5 6 7 8 9 10

Mood State 1 2 3 4 5 6 7 8 9 10

Goal _____

Workout _____

Specific Task _____

Actual Workout Time _____

Distance _____ Cadence _____

Average Heart Rate _____ Power _____

Interval 1: TIME _____ HR _____ P _____
Interval 2: TIME _____ HR _____ P _____
Interval 3: TIME _____ HR _____ P _____
Interval 4: TIME _____ HR _____ P _____
Interval 5: TIME _____ HR _____ P _____

Workout Notes _____

Personal Notes _____

Sunday ■ Date: ___ / ___ / ___

Waking Heart Rate ___

Standing Heart Rate ___

Waking Weight ___ Hours of Sleep ___

Quality of Sleep 1 2 3 4 5 6 7 8 9 10

Mood State 1 2 3 4 5 6 7 8 9 10

Goal ___

Workout ___

Specific Task ___

Actual Workout Time ___

Distance ___ Cadence ___

Average Heart Rate ___ Power ___

Interval 1: TIME ___ HR ___ P ___
Interval 2: TIME ___ HR ___ P ___
Interval 3: TIME ___ HR ___ P ___
Interval 4: TIME ___ HR ___ P ___
Interval 5: TIME ___ HR ___ P ___

Workout Notes ___

Personal Notes ___

Weekly Summary

Hours of Cycling: ___ Year-to-Date: ___

Miles/Kilometers: ___ Year-to-Date: ___

Hours of Strength Training: ___ Year-to-Date: ___

Hours of Other Activities: ___ Year-to-Date: ___

___ Year-to-Date: ___

___ Year-to-Date: ___

___ Year-to-Date: ___

Total Training Hours: ___

Number of Workouts Planned: ___

Number of Workouts Completed: ___

Average Hours of Sleep: ___

Average Quality of Sleep: ___

Average Mood State: ___

Time Spent in Heart Rate/Power Ranges:

CTS RANGES	TIME	CTS RANGES	TIME	OTHER WORKOUTS	TIME
RecoveryMiles™		SteadyState™			
FoundationMiles™		ClimbingRepeats™			
EnduranceMiles™		Max Effort			
Tempo™					

Personal Notes: ___

Weekly Strength Training Record

Exercise	Date:						Date:						Date:					
	SET 1		SET 2		SET 3		SET 1		SET 2		SET 3		SET 1		SET 2		SET 3	
	lbs.	reps	lbs.	reps	lbs.	reps	lbs.	reps	lbs.	reps	lbs.	reps	lbs.	reps	lbs.	reps	lbs.	reps

Race Results

Race #1 _____ Date: ___ / ___ / ___

Time _____ Distance _____

Goal _____

Result _____

Average Heart Rate _____ Power _____

Food/Fluid Intake _____

Personal Notes _____

_____

_____

Race #2 _____ Date: ___ / ___ / ___

Time _____ Distance _____

Goal _____

Result _____

Average Heart Rate _____ Power _____

Food/Fluid Intake _____

Personal Notes _____

_____

_____

Week # _____ Goal: _____

Monday ■ Date: ___ / ___ / ___

Waking Heart Rate _____

Standing Heart Rate _____

Waking Weight _____ Hours of Sleep _____

Quality of Sleep 1 2 3 4 5 6 7 8 9 10

Mood State 1 2 3 4 5 6 7 8 9 10

Goal _____

Workout _____

Specific Task _____

Actual Workout Time _____

Distance _____ Cadence _____

Average Heart Rate _____ Power _____

Interval 1: TIME _____ HR _____ P _____

Interval 2: TIME _____ HR _____ P _____

Interval 3: TIME _____ HR _____ P _____

Interval 4: TIME _____ HR _____ P _____

Interval 5: TIME _____ HR _____ P _____

Workout Notes _____

Personal Notes _____

Tuesday ■ Date: ___ / ___ / ___

Waking Heart Rate _____

Standing Heart Rate _____

Waking Weight _____ Hours of Sleep _____

Quality of Sleep 1 2 3 4 5 6 7 8 9 10

Mood State 1 2 3 4 5 6 7 8 9 10

Goal _____

Workout _____

Specific Task _____

Actual Workout Time _____

Distance _____ Cadence _____

Average Heart Rate _____ Power _____

Interval 1: TIME _____ HR _____ P _____

Interval 2: TIME _____ HR _____ P _____

Interval 3: TIME _____ HR _____ P _____

Interval 4: TIME _____ HR _____ P _____

Interval 5: TIME _____ HR _____ P _____

Workout Notes _____

Personal Notes _____

Wednesday ■ Date: ___ / ___ / ___

Waking Heart Rate _____

Standing Heart Rate _____

Waking Weight _____ Hours of Sleep _____

Quality of Sleep 1 2 3 4 5 6 7 8 9 10

Mood State 1 2 3 4 5 6 7 8 9 10

Goal _____

Workout _____

Specific Task _____

Actual Workout Time _____

Distance _____ Cadence _____

Average Heart Rate _____ Power _____

Interval 1: TIME _____ HR _____ P _____

Interval 2: TIME _____ HR _____ P _____

Interval 3: TIME _____ HR _____ P _____

Interval 4: TIME _____ HR _____ P _____

Interval 5: TIME _____ HR _____ P _____

Workout Notes _____

Personal Notes _____

Thursday ■ Date: ___ / ___ / ___

Waking Heart Rate _____

Standing Heart Rate _____

Waking Weight _____ Hours of Sleep _____

Quality of Sleep 1 2 3 4 5 6 7 8 9 10

Mood State 1 2 3 4 5 6 7 8 9 10

Goal _____

Workout _____

Specific Task _____

Actual Workout Time _____

Distance _____ Cadence _____

Average Heart Rate _____ Power _____

Interval 1: TIME _____ HR _____ P _____
Interval 2: TIME _____ HR _____ P _____
Interval 3: TIME _____ HR _____ P _____
Interval 4: TIME _____ HR _____ P _____
Interval 5: TIME _____ HR _____ P _____

Workout Notes _____

Personal Notes _____

Friday ■ Date: ___ / ___ / ___

Waking Heart Rate _____

Standing Heart Rate _____

Waking Weight _____ Hours of Sleep _____

Quality of Sleep 1 2 3 4 5 6 7 8 9 10

Mood State 1 2 3 4 5 6 7 8 9 10

Goal _____

Workout _____

Specific Task _____

Actual Workout Time _____

Distance _____ Cadence _____

Average Heart Rate _____ Power _____

Interval 1: TIME _____ HR _____ P _____
Interval 2: TIME _____ HR _____ P _____
Interval 3: TIME _____ HR _____ P _____
Interval 4: TIME _____ HR _____ P _____
Interval 5: TIME _____ HR _____ P _____

Workout Notes _____

Personal Notes _____

Saturday ■ Date: ___ / ___ / ___

Waking Heart Rate _____

Standing Heart Rate _____

Waking Weight _____ Hours of Sleep _____

Quality of Sleep 1 2 3 4 5 6 7 8 9 10

Mood State 1 2 3 4 5 6 7 8 9 10

Goal _____

Workout _____

Specific Task _____

Actual Workout Time _____

Distance _____ Cadence _____

Average Heart Rate _____ Power _____

Interval 1: TIME _____ HR _____ P _____
Interval 2: TIME _____ HR _____ P _____
Interval 3: TIME _____ HR _____ P _____
Interval 4: TIME _____ HR _____ P _____
Interval 5: TIME _____ HR _____ P _____

Workout Notes _____

Personal Notes _____

Sunday ■ Date: ___ / ___ / ___

Waking Heart Rate _____

Standing Heart Rate _____

Waking Weight _____ Hours of Sleep _____

Quality of Sleep 1 2 3 4 5 6 7 8 9 10

Mood State 1 2 3 4 5 6 7 8 9 10

Goal _____

Workout _____

Specific Task _____

Actual Workout Time _____

Distance _____ Cadence _____

Average Heart Rate _____ Power _____

Interval 1:	TIME	HR	P	
Interval 2:	TIME	HR	P	
Interval 3:	TIME	HR	P	
Interval 4:	TIME	HR	P	
Interval 5:	TIME	HR	P	

Workout Notes _____

Personal Notes _____

Weekly Summary

Hours of Cycling: _____ Year-to-Date: _____

Miles/Kilometers: _____ Year-to-Date: _____

Hours of Strength Training: _____ Year-to-Date: _____

Hours of Other Activities: _____ Year-to-Date: _____

_____ Year-to-Date: _____

_____ Year-to-Date: _____

Total Training Hours: _____ Year-to-Date: _____

Number of Workouts Planned: _____

Number of Workouts Completed: _____

Average Hours of Sleep: _____

Average Quality of Sleep: _____

Average Mood State: _____

Time Spent in Heart Rate/Power Ranges:

CTS RANGES	TIME	CTS RANGES	TIME	OTHER WORKOUTS	TIME
RecoveryMiles™		SteadyState™			
FoundationMiles™		ClimbingRepeats™			
EnduranceMiles™		Max Effort			
Tempo™					

Personal Notes: _____

Weekly Strength Training Record

Exercise	Date:						Date:						Date:					
	SET 1 lbs. / reps		SET 2 lbs. / reps		SET 3 lbs. / reps		SET 1 lbs. / reps		SET 2 lbs. / reps		SET 3 lbs. / reps		SET 1 lbs. / reps		SET 2 lbs. / reps		SET 3 lbs. / reps	

Race Results

Race #1_____ Date: ___/___/___

Time_____ Distance_____

Goal_____

Result_____

Average Heart Rate_____ Power_____

Food/Fluid Intake_____

Personal Notes_____

_____

_____

Race #2_____ Date: ___/___/___

Time_____ Distance_____

Goal_____

Result_____

Average Heart Rate_____ Power_____

Food/Fluid Intake_____

Personal Notes_____

_____

_____

Week # _____ Goal: _____

Monday ■ Date: ___ / ___ / ___

Waking Heart Rate _____

Standing Heart Rate _____

Waking Weight _____ Hours of Sleep _____

Quality of Sleep 1 2 3 4 5 6 7 8 9 10

Mood State 1 2 3 4 5 6 7 8 9 10

Goal _____

Workout _____

Specific Task _____

Actual Workout Time _____

Distance _____ Cadence _____ Power _____

Average Heart Rate _____

Interval 1:	TIME _____	HR _____	P _____
Interval 2:	TIME _____	HR _____	P _____
Interval 3:	TIME _____	HR _____	P _____
Interval 4:	TIME _____	HR _____	P _____
Interval 5:	TIME _____	HR _____	P _____

Workout Notes _____

Personal Notes _____

Tuesday ■ Date: ___ / ___ / ___

Waking Heart Rate _____

Standing Heart Rate _____

Waking Weight _____ Hours of Sleep _____

Quality of Sleep 1 2 3 4 5 6 7 8 9 10

Mood State 1 2 3 4 5 6 7 8 9 10

Goal _____

Workout _____

Specific Task _____

Actual Workout Time _____

Distance _____ Cadence _____ Power _____

Average Heart Rate _____

Interval 1:	TIME _____	HR _____	P _____
Interval 2:	TIME _____	HR _____	P _____
Interval 3:	TIME _____	HR _____	P _____
Interval 4:	TIME _____	HR _____	P _____
Interval 5:	TIME _____	HR _____	P _____

Workout Notes _____

Personal Notes _____

Wednesday ■ Date: ___ / ___ / ___

Waking Heart Rate _____

Standing Heart Rate _____

Waking Weight _____ Hours of Sleep _____

Quality of Sleep 1 2 3 4 5 6 7 8 9 10

Mood State 1 2 3 4 5 6 7 8 9 10

Goal _____

Workout _____

Specific Task _____

Actual Workout Time _____

Distance _____ Cadence _____ Power _____

Average Heart Rate _____

Interval 1:	TIME _____	HR _____	P _____
Interval 2:	TIME _____	HR _____	P _____
Interval 3:	TIME _____	HR _____	P _____
Interval 4:	TIME _____	HR _____	P _____
Interval 5:	TIME _____	HR _____	P _____

Workout Notes _____

Personal Notes _____

Thursday ■ Date: ___ / ___ / ___

Waking Heart Rate _____

Standing Heart Rate _____

Waking Weight _____ Hours of Sleep _____

Quality of Sleep 1 2 3 4 5 6 7 8 9 10

Mood State 1 2 3 4 5 6 7 8 9 10

Goal _____

Workout _____

Specific Task _____

Actual Workout Time _____

Distance _____ Cadence _____ Power _____

Average Heart Rate _____

Interval 1: TIME _____ HR _____ P _____
Interval 2: TIME _____ HR _____ P _____
Interval 3: TIME _____ HR _____ P _____
Interval 4: TIME _____ HR _____ P _____
Interval 5: TIME _____ HR _____ P _____

Workout Notes _____

Personal Notes _____

Friday ■ Date: ___ / ___ / ___

Waking Heart Rate _____

Standing Heart Rate _____

Waking Weight _____ Hours of Sleep _____

Quality of Sleep 1 2 3 4 5 6 7 8 9 10

Mood State 1 2 3 4 5 6 7 8 9 10

Goal _____

Workout _____

Specific Task _____

Actual Workout Time _____

Distance _____ Cadence _____ Power _____

Average Heart Rate _____

Interval 1: TIME _____ HR _____ P _____
Interval 2: TIME _____ HR _____ P _____
Interval 3: TIME _____ HR _____ P _____
Interval 4: TIME _____ HR _____ P _____
Interval 5: TIME _____ HR _____ P _____

Workout Notes _____

Personal Notes _____

Saturday ■ Date: ___ / ___ / ___

Waking Heart Rate _____

Standing Heart Rate _____

Waking Weight _____ Hours of Sleep _____

Quality of Sleep 1 2 3 4 5 6 7 8 9 10

Mood State 1 2 3 4 5 6 7 8 9 10

Goal _____

Workout _____

Specific Task _____

Actual Workout Time _____

Distance _____ Cadence _____ Power _____

Average Heart Rate _____

Interval 1: TIME _____ HR _____ P _____
Interval 2: TIME _____ HR _____ P _____
Interval 3: TIME _____ HR _____ P _____
Interval 4: TIME _____ HR _____ P _____
Interval 5: TIME _____ HR _____ P _____

Workout Notes _____

Personal Notes _____

Week #

Sunday ■ Date: ___ / ___ / ___

Waking Heart Rate ___

Standing Heart Rate ___

Waking Weight ___ Hours of Sleep ___

Quality of Sleep 1 2 3 4 5 6 7 8 9 10

Mood State 1 2 3 4 5 6 7 8 9 10

Goal ___

Workout ___

Specific Task ___

Actual Workout Time ___

Distance ___ Cadence ___

Average Heart Rate ___ Power ___

Interval 1: TIME ___ HR ___ P ___

Interval 2: TIME ___ HR ___ P ___

Interval 3: TIME ___ HR ___ P ___

Interval 4: TIME ___ HR ___ P ___

Interval 5: TIME ___ HR ___ P ___

Workout Notes ___

Personal Notes ___

Weekly Summary

Hours of Cycling: ___ Year-to-Date: ___

Miles/Kilometers: ___ Year-to-Date: ___

Hours of Strength Training: ___ Year-to-Date: ___

Hours of Other Activities: ___ Year-to-Date: ___

___ Year-to-Date: ___

Total Training Hours: ___ Year-to-Date: ___

Number of Workouts Planned: ___ Year-to-Date: ___

Number of Workouts Completed: ___

Average Hours of Sleep: ___

Average Quality of Sleep: ___

Average Mood State: ___

Time Spent in Heart Rate/Power Ranges:

CTS RANGES	TIME	CTS RANGES	TIME	OTHER WORKOUTS	TIME
RecoveryMiles™		SteadyState™			
FoundationMiles™		ClimbingRepeats™			
EnduranceMiles™		Max Effort			
Tempo™					

Personal Notes: ___

Week # Weekly Strength Training Record

Race Results

Race #1 _____ Date: ___/___/___

Time_____ Distance_____

Goal_____

Result_____

Average Heart Rate_____ Power_____

Food/Fluid Intake_____

Personal Notes_____

_____

Race #2 _____ Date: ___/___/___

Time_____ Distance_____

Goal_____

Result_____

Average Heart Rate_____ Power_____

Food/Fluid Intake_____

Personal Notes_____

_____

Exercise

Exercise	Date:						Date:						Date:					
	SET 1		SET 2		SET 3		SET 1		SET 2		SET 3		SET 1		SET 2		SET 3	
	lbs.	reps	lbs.	reps	lbs.	reps	lbs.	reps	lbs.	reps	lbs.	reps	lbs.	reps	lbs.	reps	lbs.	reps

| Week # _____ | Goal: _____ |

Monday ▪ Date: ___ / ___ / ___

Waking Heart Rate _____

Standing Heart Rate _____

Waking Weight _____ Hours of Sleep _____

Quality of Sleep 1 2 3 4 5 6 7 8 9 10

Mood State 1 2 3 4 5 6 7 8 9 10

Goal _____

Workout _____

Specific Task _____

Actual Workout Time _____

Distance _____ Cadence _____

Average Heart Rate _____ Power _____

Interval 1: TIME _____ HR _____ P. _____
Interval 2: TIME _____ HR _____ P. _____
Interval 3: TIME _____ HR _____ P. _____
Interval 4: TIME _____ HR _____ P. _____
Interval 5: TIME _____ HR _____ P. _____

Workout Notes _____

Personal Notes _____

Tuesday ▪ Date: ___ / ___ / ___

Waking Heart Rate _____

Standing Heart Rate _____

Waking Weight _____ Hours of Sleep _____

Quality of Sleep 1 2 3 4 5 6 7 8 9 10

Mood State 1 2 3 4 5 6 7 8 9 10

Goal _____

Workout _____

Specific Task _____

Actual Workout Time _____

Distance _____ Cadence _____

Average Heart Rate _____ Power _____

Interval 1: TIME _____ HR _____ P. _____
Interval 2: TIME _____ HR _____ P. _____
Interval 3: TIME _____ HR _____ P. _____
Interval 4: TIME _____ HR _____ P. _____
Interval 5: TIME _____ HR _____ P. _____

Workout Notes _____

Personal Notes _____

Wednesday ▪ Date: ___ / ___ / ___

Waking Heart Rate _____

Standing Heart Rate _____

Waking Weight _____ Hours of Sleep _____

Quality of Sleep 1 2 3 4 5 6 7 8 9 10

Mood State 1 2 3 4 5 6 7 8 9 10

Goal _____

Workout _____

Specific Task _____

Actual Workout Time _____

Distance _____ Cadence _____

Average Heart Rate _____ Power _____

Interval 1: TIME _____ HR _____ P. _____
Interval 2: TIME _____ HR _____ P. _____
Interval 3: TIME _____ HR _____ P. _____
Interval 4: TIME _____ HR _____ P. _____
Interval 5: TIME _____ HR _____ P. _____

Workout Notes _____

Personal Notes _____

Week #

Thursday ■ Date: ___ / ___ / ___

Waking Heart Rate _____

Standing Heart Rate _____

Waking Weight _____ Hours of Sleep _____

Quality of Sleep 1 2 3 4 5 6 7 8 9 10

Mood State 1 2 3 4 5 6 7 8 9 10

Goal _____

Workout _____

Specific Task _____

Actual Workout Time _____

Distance _____ Cadence _____

Average Heart Rate _____ Power _____

Interval 1: TIME _____ HR _____ P _____
Interval 2: TIME _____ HR _____ P _____
Interval 3: TIME _____ HR _____ P _____
Interval 4: TIME _____ HR _____ P _____
Interval 5: TIME _____ HR _____ P _____

Workout Notes _____

Personal Notes _____

Friday ■ Date: ___ / ___ / ___

Waking Heart Rate _____

Standing Heart Rate _____

Waking Weight _____ Hours of Sleep _____

Quality of Sleep 1 2 3 4 5 6 7 8 9 10

Mood State 1 2 3 4 5 6 7 8 9 10

Goal _____

Workout _____

Specific Task _____

Actual Workout Time _____

Distance _____ Cadence _____

Average Heart Rate _____ Power _____

Interval 1: TIME _____ HR _____ P _____
Interval 2: TIME _____ HR _____ P _____
Interval 3: TIME _____ HR _____ P _____
Interval 4: TIME _____ HR _____ P _____
Interval 5: TIME _____ HR _____ P _____

Workout Notes _____

Personal Notes _____

Saturday ■ Date: ___ / ___ / ___

Waking Heart Rate _____

Standing Heart Rate _____

Waking Weight _____ Hours of Sleep _____

Quality of Sleep 1 2 3 4 5 6 7 8 9 10

Mood State 1 2 3 4 5 6 7 8 9 10

Goal _____

Workout _____

Specific Task _____

Actual Workout Time _____

Distance _____ Cadence _____

Average Heart Rate _____ Power _____

Interval 1: TIME _____ HR _____ P _____
Interval 2: TIME _____ HR _____ P _____
Interval 3: TIME _____ HR _____ P _____
Interval 4: TIME _____ HR _____ P _____
Interval 5: TIME _____ HR _____ P _____

Workout Notes _____

Personal Notes _____

Sunday ■ Date: ___ / ___ / ___

Waking Heart Rate _____

Standing Heart Rate _____

Waking Weight _____ Hours of Sleep _____

Quality of Sleep 1 2 3 4 5 6 7 8 9 10

Mood State 1 2 3 4 5 6 7 8 9 10

Goal _____

Workout _____

Specific Task _____

Actual Workout Time _____

Distance _____ Cadence _____

Average Heart Rate _____ Power _____

Interval 1: TIME _____ HR _____ P _____

Interval 2: TIME _____ HR _____ P _____

Interval 3: TIME _____ HR _____ P _____

Interval 4: TIME _____ HR _____ P _____

Interval 5: TIME _____ HR _____ P _____

Workout Notes _____

Personal Notes _____

Weekly Summary

Hours of Cycling: _____ Year-to-Date: _____

Miles/Kilometers: _____ Year-to-Date: _____

Hours of Strength Training: _____ Year-to-Date: _____

Hours of Other Activities: _____ Year-to-Date: _____

_____ Year-to-Date: _____

Total Training Hours: _____ Year-to-Date: _____

Number of Workouts Planned: _____

Number of Workouts Completed: _____

Average Hours of Sleep: _____

Average Quality of Sleep: _____

Average Mood State: _____

Time Spent in Heart Rate/Power Ranges:

CTS RANGES	TIME	CTS RANGES	TIME	OTHER WORKOUTS	TIME
RecoveryMiles™	_____	SteadyState™	_____		_____
FoundationMiles™	_____	ClimbingRepeats™	_____		_____
EnduranceMiles™	_____	Max Effort	_____		_____
Tempo™	_____				

Personal Notes: _____

Weekly Strength Training Record

Race Results

Race #1 _____ Date: ___ / ___ / ___

Time _____ Distance _____

Goal _____

Result _____

Average Heart Rate _____ Power _____

Food/Fluid Intake _____

Personal Notes _____

_____

_____

_____

Race #2 _____ Date: ___ / ___ / ___

Time _____ Distance _____

Goal _____

Result _____

Average Heart Rate _____ Power _____

Food/Fluid Intake _____

Personal Notes _____

_____

_____

_____

Exercise	Date:						Date:						Date:					
	SET 1		SET 2		SET 3		SET 1		SET 2		SET 3		SET 1		SET 2		SET 3	
	lbs.	reps	lbs.	reps	lbs.	reps	lbs.	reps	lbs.	reps	lbs.	reps	lbs.	reps	lbs.	reps	lbs.	reps

Week # _____ Goal: _____

Monday ■ Date: ___/___/___

Waking Heart Rate _____

Standing Heart Rate _____

Waking Weight _____ Hours of Sleep _____

Quality of Sleep 1 2 3 4 5 6 7 8 9 10

Mood State 1 2 3 4 5 6 7 8 9 10

Goal _____

Workout _____

Specific Task _____

Actual Workout Time _____

Distance _____ Cadence _____

Average Heart Rate _____ Power _____

Interval 1: TIME _____ HR _____ P _____
Interval 2: TIME _____ HR _____ P _____
Interval 3: TIME _____ HR _____ P _____
Interval 4: TIME _____ HR _____ P _____
Interval 5: TIME _____ HR _____ P _____

Workout Notes _____

Personal Notes _____

Tuesday ■ Date: ___/___/___

Waking Heart Rate _____

Standing Heart Rate _____

Waking Weight _____ Hours of Sleep _____

Quality of Sleep 1 2 3 4 5 6 7 8 9 10

Mood State 1 2 3 4 5 6 7 8 9 10

Goal _____

Workout _____

Specific Task _____

Actual Workout Time _____

Distance _____ Cadence _____

Average Heart Rate _____ Power _____

Interval 1: TIME _____ HR _____ P _____
Interval 2: TIME _____ HR _____ P _____
Interval 3: TIME _____ HR _____ P _____
Interval 4: TIME _____ HR _____ P _____
Interval 5: TIME _____ HR _____ P _____

Workout Notes _____

Personal Notes _____

Wednesday ■ Date: ___/___/___

Waking Heart Rate _____

Standing Heart Rate _____

Waking Weight _____ Hours of Sleep _____

Quality of Sleep 1 2 3 4 5 6 7 8 9 10

Mood State 1 2 3 4 5 6 7 8 9 10

Goal _____

Workout _____

Specific Task _____

Actual Workout Time _____

Distance _____ Cadence _____

Average Heart Rate _____ Power _____

Interval 1: TIME _____ HR _____ P _____
Interval 2: TIME _____ HR _____ P _____
Interval 3: TIME _____ HR _____ P _____
Interval 4: TIME _____ HR _____ P _____
Interval 5: TIME _____ HR _____ P _____

Workout Notes _____

Personal Notes _____

Thursday ■ Date: ___ / ___ / ___

Waking Heart Rate ___

Standing Heart Rate ___

Waking Weight ___ Hours of Sleep ___

Quality of Sleep 1 2 3 4 5 6 7 8 9 10

Mood State 1 2 3 4 5 6 7 8 9 10

Goal ___

Workout ___

Specific Task ___

Actual Workout Time ___

Distance ___ Cadence ___

Average Heart Rate ___ Power ___

Interval 1: TIME ___ HR ___ P ___
Interval 2: TIME ___ HR ___ P ___
Interval 3: TIME ___ HR ___ P ___
Interval 4: TIME ___ HR ___ P ___
Interval 5: TIME ___ HR ___ P ___

Workout Notes ___

Personal Notes ___

Friday ■ Date: ___ / ___ / ___

Waking Heart Rate ___

Standing Heart Rate ___

Waking Weight ___ Hours of Sleep ___

Quality of Sleep 1 2 3 4 5 6 7 8 9 10

Mood State 1 2 3 4 5 6 7 8 9 10

Goal ___

Workout ___

Specific Task ___

Actual Workout Time ___

Distance ___ Cadence ___

Average Heart Rate ___ Power ___

Interval 1: TIME ___ HR ___ P ___
Interval 2: TIME ___ HR ___ P ___
Interval 3: TIME ___ HR ___ P ___
Interval 4: TIME ___ HR ___ P ___
Interval 5: TIME ___ HR ___ P ___

Workout Notes ___

Personal Notes ___

Saturday ■ Date: ___ / ___ / ___

Waking Heart Rate ___

Standing Heart Rate ___

Waking Weight ___ Hours of Sleep ___

Quality of Sleep 1 2 3 4 5 6 7 8 9 10

Mood State 1 2 3 4 5 6 7 8 9 10

Goal ___

Workout ___

Specific Task ___

Actual Workout Time ___

Distance ___ Cadence ___

Average Heart Rate ___ Power ___

Interval 1: TIME ___ HR ___ P ___
Interval 2: TIME ___ HR ___ P ___
Interval 3: TIME ___ HR ___ P ___
Interval 4: TIME ___ HR ___ P ___
Interval 5: TIME ___ HR ___ P ___

Workout Notes ___

Personal Notes ___

Week #

Sunday ■ Date: ___ / ___ / ___

Waking Heart Rate _____

Standing Heart Rate _____

Waking Weight _____ Hours of Sleep _____

Quality of Sleep 1 2 3 4 5 6 7 8 9 10

Mood State 1 2 3 4 5 6 7 8 9 10

Goal _____

Workout _____

Specific Task _____

Actual Workout Time _____

Distance _____ Cadence _____

Average Heart Rate _____ Power _____

Interval 1:	TIME ____	HR ____	P ____
Interval 2:	TIME ____	HR ____	P ____
Interval 3:	TIME ____	HR ____	P ____
Interval 4:	TIME ____	HR ____	P ____
Interval 5:	TIME ____	HR ____	P ____

Workout Notes _____

Personal Notes _____

Weekly Summary

Hours of Cycling: _____ Year-to-Date: _____

Miles/Kilometers: _____ Year-to-Date: _____

Hours of Strength Training: _____ Year-to-Date: _____

Hours of Other Activities: _____ Year-to-Date: _____

_____ Year-to-Date: _____

_____ Year-to-Date: _____

_____ Year-to-Date: _____

_____ Year-to-Date: _____

Total Training Hours: _____

Number of Workouts Planned: _____

Number of Workouts Completed: _____

Average Hours of Sleep: _____

Average Quality of Sleep: _____

Average Mood State: _____

Time Spent in Heart Rate/Power Ranges:

CTS RANGES	TIME	CTS RANGES	TIME	OTHER WORKOUTS	TIME
RecoveryMiles™	____	SteadyState™	____		____
FoundationMiles™	____	ClimbingRepeats™	____		____
EnduranceMiles™	____	Max Effort	____		____
Tempo™	____				

Personal Notes: _____

Weekly Strength Training Record

Exercise	Date:						Date:						Date:					
	SET 1		SET 2		SET 3		SET 1		SET 2		SET 3		SET 1		SET 2		SET 3	
	lbs.	reps	lbs.	reps	lbs.	reps	lbs.	reps	lbs.	reps	lbs.	reps	lbs.	reps	lbs.	reps	lbs.	reps

Race Results

Race #1 _____ Date: ___/___/___

Time _____ Distance _____

Goal _____

Result _____

Average Heart Rate _____ Power _____

Food/Fluid Intake _____

Personal Notes _____

_____

_____

Race #2 _____ Date: ___/___/___

Time _____ Distance _____

Goal _____

Result _____

Average Heart Rate _____ Power _____

Food/Fluid Intake _____

Personal Notes _____

_____

_____

Monday ■ Date: ___ / ___ / ___

Waking Heart Rate _____

Standing Heart Rate _____

Waking Weight _____ Hours of Sleep _____

Quality of Sleep 1 2 3 4 5 6 7 8 9 10

Mood State 1 2 3 4 5 6 7 8 9 10

Goal _____

Workout _____

Specific Task _____

Actual Workout Time _____

Distance _____ Cadence _____

Average Heart Rate _____ Power _____

Interval 1: TIME _____ HR _____ P _____

Interval 2: TIME _____ HR _____ P _____

Interval 3: TIME _____ HR _____ P _____

Interval 4: TIME _____ HR _____ P _____

Interval 5: TIME _____ HR _____ P _____

Workout Notes _____

Personal Notes _____

Tuesday ■ Date: ___ / ___ / ___

Waking Heart Rate _____

Standing Heart Rate _____

Waking Weight _____ Hours of Sleep _____

Quality of Sleep 1 2 3 4 5 6 7 8 9 10

Mood State 1 2 3 4 5 6 7 8 9 10

Goal _____

Workout _____

Specific Task _____

Actual Workout Time _____

Distance _____ Cadence _____

Average Heart Rate _____ Power _____

Interval 1: TIME _____ HR _____ P _____

Interval 2: TIME _____ HR _____ P _____

Interval 3: TIME _____ HR _____ P _____

Interval 4: TIME _____ HR _____ P _____

Interval 5: TIME _____ HR _____ P _____

Workout Notes _____

Personal Notes _____

Wednesday ■ Date: ___ / ___ / ___

Waking Heart Rate _____

Standing Heart Rate _____

Waking Weight _____ Hours of Sleep _____

Quality of Sleep 1 2 3 4 5 6 7 8 9 10

Mood State 1 2 3 4 5 6 7 8 9 10

Goal _____

Workout _____

Specific Task _____

Actual Workout Time _____

Distance _____ Cadence _____

Average Heart Rate _____ Power _____

Interval 1: TIME _____ HR _____ P _____

Interval 2: TIME _____ HR _____ P _____

Interval 3: TIME _____ HR _____ P _____

Interval 4: TIME _____ HR _____ P _____

Interval 5: TIME _____ HR _____ P _____

Workout Notes _____

Personal Notes _____

Thursday ■ Date: ___ / ___ / ___

Waking Heart Rate _____

Standing Heart Rate _____

Waking Weight _____ Hours of Sleep _____

Quality of Sleep 1 2 3 4 5 6 7 8 9 10

Mood State 1 2 3 4 5 6 7 8 9 10

Goal _____

Workout _____

Specific Task _____

Actual Workout Time _____

Distance _____ Cadence _____

Average Heart Rate _____ Power _____

Interval 1: TIME _____ HR _____ P _____

Interval 2: TIME _____ HR _____ P _____

Interval 3: TIME _____ HR _____ P _____

Interval 4: TIME _____ HR _____ P _____

Interval 5: TIME _____ HR _____ P _____

Workout Notes _____

Personal Notes _____

Friday ■ Date: ___ / ___ / ___

Waking Heart Rate _____

Standing Heart Rate _____

Waking Weight _____ Hours of Sleep _____

Quality of Sleep 1 2 3 4 5 6 7 8 9 10

Mood State 1 2 3 4 5 6 7 8 9 10

Goal _____

Workout _____

Specific Task _____

Actual Workout Time _____

Distance _____ Cadence _____

Average Heart Rate _____ Power _____

Interval 1: TIME _____ HR _____ P _____

Interval 2: TIME _____ HR _____ P _____

Interval 3: TIME _____ HR _____ P _____

Interval 4: TIME _____ HR _____ P _____

Interval 5: TIME _____ HR _____ P _____

Workout Notes _____

Personal Notes _____

Saturday ■ Date: ___ / ___ / ___

Waking Heart Rate _____

Standing Heart Rate _____

Waking Weight _____ Hours of Sleep _____

Quality of Sleep 1 2 3 4 5 6 7 8 9 10

Mood State 1 2 3 4 5 6 7 8 9 10

Goal _____

Workout _____

Specific Task _____

Actual Workout Time _____

Distance _____ Cadence _____

Average Heart Rate _____ Power _____

Interval 1: TIME _____ HR _____ P _____

Interval 2: TIME _____ HR _____ P _____

Interval 3: TIME _____ HR _____ P _____

Interval 4: TIME _____ HR _____ P _____

Interval 5: TIME _____ HR _____ P _____

Workout Notes _____

Personal Notes _____

Sunday ■ Date: ___ / ___ / ___

Waking Heart Rate ___

Standing Heart Rate ___

Waking Weight ___ Hours of Sleep ___

Quality of Sleep 1 2 3 4 5 6 7 8 9 10

Mood State 1 2 3 4 5 6 7 8 9 10

Goal ___

Workout ___

Specific Task ___

Actual Workout Time ___

Distance ___ Cadence ___

Average Heart Rate ___ Power ___

Interval 1: TIME ___ HR ___ P ___

Interval 2: TIME ___ HR ___ P ___

Interval 3: TIME ___ HR ___ P ___

Interval 4: TIME ___ HR ___ P ___

Interval 5: TIME ___ HR ___ P ___

Workout Notes ___

Personal Notes ___

Weekly Summary

Hours of Cycling: ___ Year-to-Date: ___

Miles/Kilometers: ___ Year-to-Date: ___

Hours of Strength Training: ___ Year-to-Date: ___

Hours of Other Activities: ___ Year-to-Date: ___

___ Year-to-Date: ___

Total Training Hours: ___ Year-to-Date: ___

Number of Workouts Planned: ___ Year-to-Date: ___

Number of Workouts Completed: ___

Average Hours of Sleep: ___

Average Quality of Sleep: ___

Average Mood State: ___

Time Spent in Heart Rate/Power Ranges:

CTS RANGES	TIME	CTS RANGES	TIME	OTHER WORKOUTS	TIME
RecoveryMiles™		SteadyState™			
FoundationMiles™		ClimbingRepeats™			
EnduranceMiles™		Max Effort			
Tempo™					

Personal Notes: ___

Weekly Strength Training Record

Race Results

Exercise	Date:						Date:					
	SET 1		SET 2		SET 3		SET 1		SET 2		SET 3	
	lbs.	reps	lbs.	reps	lbs.	reps	lbs.	reps	lbs.	reps	lbs.	reps

Race #1   Date: __ / __ / __

Time _____ Distance _____

Goal _____

Result _____

Average Heart Rate _____ Power _____

Food/Fluid Intake _____

Personal Notes _____

Race #2   Date: __ / __ / __

Time _____ Distance _____

Goal _____

Result _____

Average Heart Rate _____ Power _____

Food/Fluid Intake _____

Personal Notes _____

Week # _____ **Goal:** _____

Monday ■ Date: ___ / ___ / ___

Waking Heart Rate _____
Standing Heart Rate _____
Waking Weight _____ Hours of Sleep _____
Quality of Sleep   1 2 3 4 5 6 7 8 9 10

Mood State   1 2 3 4 5 6 7 8 9 10

Goal _____
Workout _____
Specific Task _____
Actual Workout Time _____
Distance _____ Cadence _____
Average Heart Rate _____ Power _____

Interval 1: TIME _____ HR _____ P _____
Interval 2: TIME _____ HR _____ P _____
Interval 3: TIME _____ HR _____ P _____
Interval 4: TIME _____ HR _____ P _____
Interval 5: TIME _____ HR _____ P _____

Workout Notes _____
_____
_____

Personal Notes _____
_____
_____

Tuesday ■ Date: ___ / ___ / ___

Waking Heart Rate _____
Standing Heart Rate _____
Waking Weight _____ Hours of Sleep _____
Quality of Sleep   1 2 3 4 5 6 7 8 9 10

Mood State   1 2 3 4 5 6 7 8 9 10

Goal _____
Workout _____
Specific Task _____
Actual Workout Time _____
Distance _____ Cadence _____
Average Heart Rate _____ Power _____

Interval 1: TIME _____ HR _____ P _____
Interval 2: TIME _____ HR _____ P _____
Interval 3: TIME _____ HR _____ P _____
Interval 4: TIME _____ HR _____ P _____
Interval 5: TIME _____ HR _____ P _____

Workout Notes _____
_____
_____

Personal Notes _____
_____
_____

Wednesday ■ Date: ___ / ___ / ___

Waking Heart Rate _____
Standing Heart Rate _____
Waking Weight _____ Hours of Sleep _____
Quality of Sleep   1 2 3 4 5 6 7 8 9 10

Mood State   1 2 3 4 5 6 7 8 9 10

Goal _____
Workout _____
Specific Task _____
Actual Workout Time _____
Distance _____ Cadence _____
Average Heart Rate _____ Power _____

Interval 1: TIME _____ HR _____ P _____
Interval 2: TIME _____ HR _____ P _____
Interval 3: TIME _____ HR _____ P _____
Interval 4: TIME _____ HR _____ P _____
Interval 5: TIME _____ HR _____ P _____

Workout Notes _____
_____
_____

Personal Notes _____
_____
_____

Thursday ■ Date: ___ / ___ / ___

Waking Heart Rate _____

Standing Heart Rate _____

Waking Weight _____ Hours of Sleep _____

Quality of Sleep   1 2 3 4 5 6 7 8 9 10

Mood State   1 2 3 4 5 6 7 8 9 10 _____

Goal _____

Workout _____

Specific Task _____

Actual Workout Time _____

Distance _____ Cadence _____

Average Heart Rate _____ Power _____

Interval 1: TIME _____ HR _____ P _____

Interval 2: TIME _____ HR _____ P _____

Interval 3: TIME _____ HR _____ P _____

Interval 4: TIME _____ HR _____ P _____

Interval 5: TIME _____ HR _____ P _____

Workout Notes _____

Personal Notes _____

Friday ■ Date: ___ / ___ / ___

Waking Heart Rate _____

Standing Heart Rate _____

Waking Weight _____ Hours of Sleep _____

Quality of Sleep   1 2 3 4 5 6 7 8 9 10

Mood State   1 2 3 4 5 6 7 8 9 10 _____

Goal _____

Workout _____

Specific Task _____

Actual Workout Time _____

Distance _____ Cadence _____

Average Heart Rate _____ Power _____

Interval 1: TIME _____ HR _____ P _____

Interval 2: TIME _____ HR _____ P _____

Interval 3: TIME _____ HR _____ P _____

Interval 4: TIME _____ HR _____ P _____

Interval 5: TIME _____ HR _____ P _____

Workout Notes _____

Personal Notes _____

Saturday ■ Date: ___ / ___ / ___

Waking Heart Rate _____

Standing Heart Rate _____

Waking Weight _____ Hours of Sleep _____

Quality of Sleep   1 2 3 4 5 6 7 8 9 10

Mood State   1 2 3 4 5 6 7 8 9 10 _____

Goal _____

Workout _____

Specific Task _____

Actual Workout Time _____

Distance _____ Cadence _____

Average Heart Rate _____ Power _____

Interval 1: TIME _____ HR _____ P _____

Interval 2: TIME _____ HR _____ P _____

Interval 3: TIME _____ HR _____ P _____

Interval 4: TIME _____ HR _____ P _____

Interval 5: TIME _____ HR _____ P _____

Workout Notes _____

Personal Notes _____

Sunday ■ Date: ___ / ___ / ___

Waking Heart Rate _____

Standing Heart Rate _____

Waking Weight_____ Hours of Sleep _____

Quality of Sleep   1 2 3 4 5 6 7 8 9 10

Mood State   1 2 3 4 5 6 7 8 9 10

Goal _____

Workout _____

Specific Task _____

Actual Workout Time_____

Distance _____ Cadence _____

Average Heart Rate _____ Power _____

Interval 1:   TIME _____ HR _____ P _____

Interval 2:   TIME _____ HR _____ P _____

Interval 3:   TIME _____ HR _____ P _____

Interval 4:   TIME _____ HR _____ P _____

Interval 5:   TIME _____ HR _____ P _____

Workout Notes _____

Personal Notes _____

Weekly Summary

Hours of Cycling: _____ Year-to-Date: _____

Miles/Kilometers: _____ Year-to-Date: _____

Hours of Strength Training: _____ Year-to-Date: _____

Hours of Other Activities: _____

_____ Year-to-Date: _____

_____ Year-to-Date: _____

Total Training Hours: _____ Year-to-Date: _____

Number of Workouts Planned: _____ Year-to-Date: _____

Number of Workouts Completed: _____

Average Hours of Sleep: _____

Average Quality of Sleep: _____

Average Mood State: _____

Time Spent in Heart Rate/Power Ranges:

CTS RANGES	TIME	CTS RANGES	TIME	OTHER WORKOUTS	TIME
RecoveryMiles™		SteadyState™			
FoundationMiles™		ClimbingRepeats™			
EnduranceMiles™		Max Effort			
Tempo™					

Personal Notes: _____

Weekly Strength Training Record

Exercise	Date:						Date:						Date:					
	SET 1		SET 2		SET 3		SET 1		SET 2		SET 3		SET 1		SET 2		SET 3	
	lbs.	reps	lbs.	reps	lbs.	reps	lbs.	reps	lbs.	reps	lbs.	reps	lbs.	reps	lbs.	reps	lbs.	reps

Race Results

Race #1 _____ Date: __ / __ / __

Time _____ Distance _____

Goal _____

Result _____

Average Heart Rate _____ Power _____

Food/Fluid Intake _____

Personal Notes _____

_____

_____

Race #2 _____ Date: __ / __ / __

Time _____ Distance _____

Goal _____

Result _____

Average Heart Rate _____ Power _____

Food/Fluid Intake _____

Personal Notes _____

_____

_____

Monday ■ Date: ____ / ____ / ____

Waking Heart Rate _____

Standing Heart Rate _____

Waking Weight _____ Hours of Sleep _____

Quality of Sleep 1 2 3 4 5 6 7 8 9 10

Mood State 1 2 3 4 5 6 7 8 9 10

Goal _____

Workout _____

Specific Task _____

Actual Workout Time _____

Distance _____ Cadence _____

Average Heart Rate _____ Power _____

Interval 1: TIME _____ HR _____ P_____
Interval 2: TIME _____ HR _____ P_____
Interval 3: TIME _____ HR _____ P_____
Interval 4: TIME _____ HR _____ P_____
Interval 5: TIME _____ HR _____ P_____

Workout Notes _____

Personal Notes _____

Tuesday ■ Date: ____ / ____ / ____

Waking Heart Rate _____

Standing Heart Rate _____

Waking Weight _____ Hours of Sleep _____

Quality of Sleep 1 2 3 4 5 6 7 8 9 10

Mood State 1 2 3 4 5 6 7 8 9 10

Goal _____

Workout _____

Specific Task _____

Actual Workout Time _____

Distance _____ Cadence _____

Average Heart Rate _____ Power _____

Interval 1: TIME _____ HR _____ P_____
Interval 2: TIME _____ HR _____ P_____
Interval 3: TIME _____ HR _____ P_____
Interval 4: TIME _____ HR _____ P_____
Interval 5: TIME _____ HR _____ P_____

Workout Notes _____

Personal Notes _____

Wednesday ■ Date: ____ / ____ / ____

Waking Heart Rate _____

Standing Heart Rate _____

Waking Weight _____ Hours of Sleep _____

Quality of Sleep 1 2 3 4 5 6 7 8 9 10

Mood State 1 2 3 4 5 6 7 8 9 10

Goal _____

Workout _____

Specific Task _____

Actual Workout Time _____

Distance _____ Cadence _____

Average Heart Rate _____ Power _____

Interval 1: TIME _____ HR _____ P_____
Interval 2: TIME _____ HR _____ P_____
Interval 3: TIME _____ HR _____ P_____
Interval 4: TIME _____ HR _____ P_____
Interval 5: TIME _____ HR _____ P_____

Workout Notes _____

Personal Notes _____

Thursday ▪ Date: ___ / ___ / ___

Waking Heart Rate _____

Standing Heart Rate _____

Waking Weight _____ Hours of Sleep _____

Quality of Sleep 1 2 3 4 5 6 7 8 9 10

Mood State 1 2 3 4 5 6 7 8 9 10

Goal _____

Workout _____

Specific Task _____

Actual Workout Time _____

Distance _____ Cadence _____

Average Heart Rate _____ Power _____

Interval 1: TIME _____ HR _____ P _____
Interval 2: TIME _____ HR _____ P _____
Interval 3: TIME _____ HR _____ P _____
Interval 4: TIME _____ HR _____ P _____
Interval 5: TIME _____ HR _____ P _____

Workout Notes _____

Personal Notes _____

Friday ▪ Date: ___ / ___ / ___

Waking Heart Rate _____

Standing Heart Rate _____

Waking Weight _____ Hours of Sleep _____

Quality of Sleep 1 2 3 4 5 6 7 8 9 10

Mood State 1 2 3 4 5 6 7 8 9 10

Goal _____

Workout _____

Specific Task _____

Actual Workout Time _____

Distance _____ Cadence _____

Average Heart Rate _____ Power _____

Interval 1: TIME _____ HR _____ P _____
Interval 2: TIME _____ HR _____ P _____
Interval 3: TIME _____ HR _____ P _____
Interval 4: TIME _____ HR _____ P _____
Interval 5: TIME _____ HR _____ P _____

Workout Notes _____

Personal Notes _____

Saturday ▪ Date: ___ / ___ / ___

Waking Heart Rate _____

Standing Heart Rate _____

Waking Weight _____ Hours of Sleep _____

Quality of Sleep 1 2 3 4 5 6 7 8 9 10

Mood State 1 2 3 4 5 6 7 8 9 10

Goal _____

Workout _____

Specific Task _____

Actual Workout Time _____

Distance _____ Cadence _____

Average Heart Rate _____ Power _____

Interval 1: TIME _____ HR _____ P _____
Interval 2: TIME _____ HR _____ P _____
Interval 3: TIME _____ HR _____ P _____
Interval 4: TIME _____ HR _____ P _____
Interval 5: TIME _____ HR _____ P _____

Workout Notes _____

Personal Notes _____

Week #

Sunday ■ Date: ___/___/___

Waking Heart Rate _____

Standing Heart Rate _____

Waking Weight _____ Hours of Sleep _____

Quality of Sleep   1 2 3 4 5 6 7 8 9 10

Mood State   1 2 3 4 5 6 7 8 9 10

Goal _____

Workout _____

Specific Task _____

Actual Workout Time _____

Distance _____ Cadence _____

Average Heart Rate _____ Power _____

Interval 1: TIME _____ HR _____ P _____
Interval 2: TIME _____ HR _____ P _____
Interval 3: TIME _____ HR _____ P _____
Interval 4: TIME _____ HR _____ P _____
Interval 5: TIME _____ HR _____ P _____

Workout Notes _____

Personal Notes _____

Weekly Summary

Hours of Cycling: _____ Year-to-Date: _____

Miles/Kilometers: _____ Year-to-Date: _____

Hours of Strength Training: _____ Year-to-Date: _____

Hours of Other Activities: _____

_____ Year-to-Date: _____

_____ Year-to-Date: _____

_____ Year-to-Date: _____

Total Training Hours: _____

Number of Workouts Planned: _____

Number of Workouts Completed: _____

Average Hours of Sleep: _____

Average Quality of Sleep: _____

Average Mood State: _____

Time Spent in Heart Rate/Power Ranges:

CTS RANGES	TIME	CTS RANGES	TIME	OTHER WORKOUTS	TIME
RecoveryMiles™		SteadyState™			
FoundationMiles™		ClimbingRepeats™			
EnduranceMiles™		Max Effort			
Tempo™					

Personal Notes: _____

Race Results

Race #1 _____ Date: ___ / ___ / ___

Time _____ Distance _____

Goal _____

Result _____

Average Heart Rate _____ Power _____

Food/Fluid Intake _____

Personal Notes _____

_____

_____

Race #2 _____ Date: ___ / ___ / ___

Time _____ Distance _____

Goal _____

Result _____

Average Heart Rate _____ Power _____

Food/Fluid Intake _____

Personal Notes _____

_____

_____

Week # _____

Weekly Strength Training Record

Exercise	Date:						Date:						Date:					
	SET 1		SET 2		SET 3		SET 1		SET 2		SET 3		SET 1		SET 2		SET 3	
	lbs.	reps	lbs.	reps	lbs.	reps	lbs.	reps	lbs.	reps	lbs.	reps	lbs.	reps	lbs.	reps	lbs.	reps

Week # _____   Goal: _____

Monday ■ Date: ___ / ___ / ___

Waking Heart Rate _____

Standing Heart Rate _____

Waking Weight _____ Hours of Sleep _____

Quality of Sleep   1 2 3 4 5 6 7 8 9 10

Mood State   1 2 3 4 5 6 7 8 9 10

Goal _____

Workout _____

Specific Task _____

Actual Workout Time _____

Distance _____ Cadence _____

Average Heart Rate _____ Power _____

Interval 1: TIME _____ HR _____ P _____
Interval 2: TIME _____ HR _____ P _____
Interval 3: TIME _____ HR _____ P _____
Interval 4: TIME _____ HR _____ P _____
Interval 5: TIME _____ HR _____ P _____

Workout Notes _____
_____

Personal Notes _____
_____

Tuesday ■ Date: ___ / ___ / ___

Waking Heart Rate _____

Standing Heart Rate _____

Waking Weight _____ Hours of Sleep _____

Quality of Sleep   1 2 3 4 5 6 7 8 9 10

Mood State   1 2 3 4 5 6 7 8 9 10

Goal _____

Workout _____

Specific Task _____

Actual Workout Time _____

Distance _____ Cadence _____

Average Heart Rate _____ Power _____

Interval 1: TIME _____ HR _____ P _____
Interval 2: TIME _____ HR _____ P _____
Interval 3: TIME _____ HR _____ P _____
Interval 4: TIME _____ HR _____ P _____
Interval 5: TIME _____ HR _____ P _____

Workout Notes _____
_____

Personal Notes _____
_____

Wednesday ■ Date: ___ / ___ / ___

Waking Heart Rate _____

Standing Heart Rate _____

Waking Weight _____ Hours of Sleep _____

Quality of Sleep   1 2 3 4 5 6 7 8 9 10

Mood State   1 2 3 4 5 6 7 8 9 10

Goal _____

Workout _____

Specific Task _____

Actual Workout Time _____

Distance _____ Cadence _____

Average Heart Rate _____ Power _____

Interval 1: TIME _____ HR _____ P _____
Interval 2: TIME _____ HR _____ P _____
Interval 3: TIME _____ HR _____ P _____
Interval 4: TIME _____ HR _____ P _____
Interval 5: TIME _____ HR _____ P _____

Workout Notes _____

Personal Notes _____

Thursday ■ Date: ___ / ___ / ___

Waking Heart Rate _____

Standing Heart Rate _____

Waking Weight _____ Hours of Sleep _____

Quality of Sleep 1 2 3 4 5 6 7 8 9 10

Mood State 1 2 3 4 5 6 7 8 9 10

Goal _____

Workout _____

Specific Task _____

Actual Workout Time _____

Distance _____ Cadence _____

Average Heart Rate _____ Power _____

Interval 1: TIME _____ HR _____ P _____

Interval 2: TIME _____ HR _____ P _____

Interval 3: TIME _____ HR _____ P _____

Interval 4: TIME _____ HR _____ P _____

Interval 5: TIME _____ HR _____ P _____

Workout Notes _____

Personal Notes _____

Friday ■ Date: ___ / ___ / ___

Waking Heart Rate _____

Standing Heart Rate _____

Waking Weight _____ Hours of Sleep _____

Quality of Sleep 1 2 3 4 5 6 7 8 9 10

Mood State 1 2 3 4 5 6 7 8 9 10

Goal _____

Workout _____

Specific Task _____

Actual Workout Time _____

Distance _____ Cadence _____

Average Heart Rate _____ Power _____

Interval 1: TIME _____ HR _____ P _____

Interval 2: TIME _____ HR _____ P _____

Interval 3: TIME _____ HR _____ P _____

Interval 4: TIME _____ HR _____ P _____

Interval 5: TIME _____ HR _____ P _____

Workout Notes _____

Personal Notes _____

Saturday ■ Date: ___ / ___ / ___

Waking Heart Rate _____

Standing Heart Rate _____

Waking Weight _____ Hours of Sleep _____

Quality of Sleep 1 2 3 4 5 6 7 8 9 10

Mood State 1 2 3 4 5 6 7 8 9 10

Goal _____

Workout _____

Specific Task _____

Actual Workout Time _____

Distance _____ Cadence _____

Average Heart Rate _____ Power _____

Interval 1: TIME _____ HR _____ P _____

Interval 2: TIME _____ HR _____ P _____

Interval 3: TIME _____ HR _____ P _____

Interval 4: TIME _____ HR _____ P _____

Interval 5: TIME _____ HR _____ P _____

Workout Notes _____

Personal Notes _____

Week #

Sunday ■ Date: ___ / ___ / ___

Waking Heart Rate ___

Standing Heart Rate ___

Waking Weight ___ Hours of Sleep ___

Quality of Sleep 1 2 3 4 5 6 7 8 9 10

Mood State 1 2 3 4 5 6 7 8 9 10

Goal ___

Workout ___

Specific Task ___

Actual Workout Time ___

Distance ___ Cadence ___

Average Heart Rate ___ Power ___

Interval 1: TIME ___ HR ___ P ___
Interval 2: TIME ___ HR ___ P ___
Interval 3: TIME ___ HR ___ P ___
Interval 4: TIME ___ HR ___ P ___
Interval 5: TIME ___ HR ___ P ___

Workout Notes ___

Personal Notes ___

Weekly Summary

Hours of Cycling: ___ Year-to-Date: ___

Miles/Kilometers: ___ Year-to-Date: ___

Hours of Strength Training: ___ Year-to-Date: ___

Hours of Other Activities: ___ Year-to-Date: ___

___ Year-to-Date: ___

Total Training Hours: ___ Year-to-Date: ___

Number of Workouts Planned: ___ Year-to-Date: ___

Number of Workouts Completed: ___

Average Hours of Sleep: ___

Average Quality of Sleep: ___

Average Mood State: ___

Time Spent in Heart Rate/Power Ranges:

CTS RANGES	TIME	CTS RANGES	TIME	OTHER WORKOUTS	TIME
RecoveryMiles™		SteadyState™			
FoundationMiles™		ClimbingRepeats™			
EnduranceMiles™		Max Effort			
Tempo™					

Personal Notes: ___

Weekly Strength Training Record

Exercise	Date:						Date:						Date:					
	SET 1		SET 2		SET 3		SET 1		SET 2		SET 3		SET 1		SET 2		SET 3	
	lbs.	reps	lbs.	reps	lbs.	reps	lbs.	reps	lbs.	reps	lbs.	reps	lbs.	reps	lbs.	reps	lbs.	reps

Race Results

Race #1 _____ Date: __ / __ / __

Time _____ Distance _____

Goal _____

Result _____

Average Heart Rate _____ Power _____

Food/Fluid Intake _____

Personal Notes _____

_____

_____

Race #2 _____ Date: __ / __ / __

Time _____ Distance _____

Goal _____

Result _____

Average Heart Rate _____ Power _____

Food/Fluid Intake _____

Personal Notes _____

_____

_____

Monday ■ Date: ___ / ___ / ___

Waking Heart Rate _____

Standing Heart Rate _____

Waking Weight _____ Hours of Sleep _____

Quality of Sleep 1 2 3 4 5 6 7 8 9 10

Mood State 1 2 3 4 5 6 7 8 9 10

Goal _____

Workout _____

Specific Task _____

Actual Workout Time _____

Distance _____ Cadence _____

Average Heart Rate _____ Power _____

Interval 1:	TIME _____	HR _____	P _____
Interval 2:	TIME _____	HR _____	P _____
Interval 3:	TIME _____	HR _____	P _____
Interval 4:	TIME _____	HR _____	P _____
Interval 5:	TIME _____	HR _____	P _____

Workout Notes _____

Personal Notes _____

Tuesday ■ Date: ___ / ___ / ___

Waking Heart Rate _____

Standing Heart Rate _____

Waking Weight _____ Hours of Sleep _____

Quality of Sleep 1 2 3 4 5 6 7 8 9 10

Mood State 1 2 3 4 5 6 7 8 9 10

Goal _____

Workout _____

Specific Task _____

Actual Workout Time _____

Distance _____ Cadence _____

Average Heart Rate _____ Power _____

Interval 1:	TIME _____	HR _____	P _____
Interval 2:	TIME _____	HR _____	P _____
Interval 3:	TIME _____	HR _____	P _____
Interval 4:	TIME _____	HR _____	P _____
Interval 5:	TIME _____	HR _____	P _____

Workout Notes _____

Personal Notes _____

Wednesday ■ Date: ___ / ___ / ___

Waking Heart Rate _____

Standing Heart Rate _____

Waking Weight _____ Hours of Sleep _____

Quality of Sleep 1 2 3 4 5 6 7 8 9 10

Mood State 1 2 3 4 5 6 7 8 9 10

Goal _____

Workout _____

Specific Task _____

Actual Workout Time _____

Distance _____ Cadence _____

Average Heart Rate _____ Power _____

Interval 1:	TIME _____	HR _____	P _____
Interval 2:	TIME _____	HR _____	P _____
Interval 3:	TIME _____	HR _____	P _____
Interval 4:	TIME _____	HR _____	P _____
Interval 5:	TIME _____	HR _____	P _____

Workout Notes _____

Personal Notes _____

Week #

Thursday ▪ Date: ___/___/___

Waking Heart Rate _____
Standing Heart Rate _____
Waking Weight _____ Hours of Sleep _____
Quality of Sleep 1 2 3 4 5 6 7 8 9 10

Mood State 1 2 3 4 5 6 7 8 9 10

Goal _____
Workout _____
Specific Task _____
Actual Workout Time _____
Distance _____ Cadence _____
Average Heart Rate _____ Power _____

Interval 1: TIME _____ HR _____ P _____
Interval 2: TIME _____ HR _____ P _____
Interval 3: TIME _____ HR _____ P _____
Interval 4: TIME _____ HR _____ P _____
Interval 5: TIME _____ HR _____ P _____

Workout Notes _____

Personal Notes _____

Friday ▪ Date: ___/___/___

Waking Heart Rate _____
Standing Heart Rate _____
Waking Weight _____ Hours of Sleep _____
Quality of Sleep 1 2 3 4 5 6 7 8 9 10

Mood State 1 2 3 4 5 6 7 8 9 10

Goal _____
Workout _____
Specific Task _____
Actual Workout Time _____
Distance _____ Cadence _____
Average Heart Rate _____ Power _____

Interval 1: TIME _____ HR _____ P _____
Interval 2: TIME _____ HR _____ P _____
Interval 3: TIME _____ HR _____ P _____
Interval 4: TIME _____ HR _____ P _____
Interval 5: TIME _____ HR _____ P _____

Workout Notes _____

Personal Notes _____

Saturday ▪ Date: ___/___/___

Waking Heart Rate _____
Standing Heart Rate _____
Waking Weight _____ Hours of Sleep _____
Quality of Sleep 1 2 3 4 5 6 7 8 9 10

Mood State 1 2 3 4 5 6 7 8 9 10

Goal _____
Workout _____
Specific Task _____
Actual Workout Time _____
Distance _____ Cadence _____
Average Heart Rate _____ Power _____

Interval 1: TIME _____ HR _____ P _____
Interval 2: TIME _____ HR _____ P _____
Interval 3: TIME _____ HR _____ P _____
Interval 4: TIME _____ HR _____ P _____
Interval 5: TIME _____ HR _____ P _____

Workout Notes _____

Personal Notes _____

Week #

Sunday ■ Date: ___ / ___ / ___

Waking Heart Rate _____

Standing Heart Rate _____

Waking Weight _____ Hours of Sleep _____

Quality of Sleep 1 2 3 4 5 6 7 8 9 10

Mood State 1 2 3 4 5 6 7 8 9 10

Goal _____

Workout _____

Specific Task _____

Actual Workout Time _____

Distance _____ Cadence _____

Average Heart Rate _____ Power _____

Interval 1: TIME _____ HR _____ P _____

Interval 2: TIME _____ HR _____ P _____

Interval 3: TIME _____ HR _____ P _____

Interval 4: TIME _____ HR _____ P _____

Interval 5: TIME _____ HR _____ P _____

Workout Notes _____

Personal Notes _____

Weekly Summary

Hours of Cycling: _____ Year-to-Date: _____

Miles/Kilometers: _____ Year-to-Date: _____

Hours of Strength Training: _____ Year-to-Date: _____

Hours of Other Activities: _____

_____ Year-to-Date: _____

_____ Year-to-Date: _____

_____ Year-to-Date: _____

Total Training Hours: _____ Year-to-Date: _____

Number of Workouts Planned: _____

Number of Workouts Completed: _____

Average Hours of Sleep: _____

Average Quality of Sleep: _____

Average Mood State: _____

Time Spent in Heart Rate/Power Ranges:

CTS RANGES	TIME	CTS RANGES	TIME	OTHER WORKOUTS	TIME
RecoveryMiles™		SteadyState™			
FoundationMiles™		ClimbingRepeats™			
EnduranceMiles™		Max Effort			
Tempo™					

Personal Notes: _____

Weekly Strength Training Record

Race Results

Race #1 _____ Date: ___/___/___

Time _____ Distance _____

Goal _____

Result _____

Average Heart Rate _____ Power _____

Food/Fluid Intake _____

Personal Notes _____

_____

_____

Race #2 _____ Date: ___/___/___

Time _____ Distance _____

Goal _____

Result _____

Average Heart Rate _____ Power _____

Food/Fluid Intake _____

Personal Notes _____

_____

_____

Exercise	Date:						Date:						Date:					
	SET 1		SET 2		SET 3		SET 1		SET 2		SET 3		SET 1		SET 2		SET 3	
	lbs.	reps	lbs.	reps	lbs.	reps	lbs.	reps	lbs.	reps	lbs.	reps	lbs.	reps	lbs.	reps	lbs.	reps

Week # _____   Goal: _____

Monday ■ Date: ___/___/___

Waking Heart Rate _____

Standing Heart Rate _____

Waking Weight _____   Hours of Sleep _____

Quality of Sleep   1 2 3 4 5 6 7 8 9 10

Mood State   1 2 3 4 5 6 7 8 9 10

Goal _____

Workout _____

Specific Task _____

Actual Workout Time _____

Distance _____   Cadence _____

Average Heart Rate _____   Power _____

Interval 1:   TIME _____   HR _____   P _____
Interval 2:   TIME _____   HR _____   P _____
Interval 3:   TIME _____   HR _____   P _____
Interval 4:   TIME _____   HR _____   P _____
Interval 5:   TIME _____   HR _____   P _____

Workout Notes _____

Personal Notes _____

Tuesday ■ Date: ___/___/___

Waking Heart Rate _____

Standing Heart Rate _____

Waking Weight _____   Hours of Sleep _____

Quality of Sleep   1 2 3 4 5 6 7 8 9 10

Mood State   1 2 3 4 5 6 7 8 9 10

Goal _____

Workout _____

Specific Task _____

Actual Workout Time _____

Distance _____   Cadence _____

Average Heart Rate _____   Power _____

Interval 1:   TIME _____   HR _____   P _____
Interval 2:   TIME _____   HR _____   P _____
Interval 3:   TIME _____   HR _____   P _____
Interval 4:   TIME _____   HR _____   P _____
Interval 5:   TIME _____   HR _____   P _____

Workout Notes _____

Personal Notes _____

Wednesday ■ Date: ___/___/___

Waking Heart Rate _____

Standing Heart Rate _____

Waking Weight _____   Hours of Sleep _____

Quality of Sleep   1 2 3 4 5 6 7 8 9 10

Mood State   1 2 3 4 5 6 7 8 9 10

Goal _____

Workout _____

Specific Task _____

Actual Workout Time _____

Distance _____   Cadence _____

Average Heart Rate _____   Power _____

Interval 1:   TIME _____   HR _____   P _____
Interval 2:   TIME _____   HR _____   P _____
Interval 3:   TIME _____   HR _____   P _____
Interval 4:   TIME _____   HR _____   P _____
Interval 5:   TIME _____   HR _____   P _____

Workout Notes _____

Personal Notes _____

Thursday ■ Date: ___ / ___ / ___

Waking Heart Rate _____

Standing Heart Rate _____

Waking Weight _____ Hours of Sleep _____

Quality of Sleep 1 2 3 4 5 6 7 8 9 10

Mood State 1 2 3 4 5 6 7 8 9 10

Goal _____

Workout _____

Specific Task _____

Actual Workout Time _____

Distance _____ Cadence _____

Average Heart Rate _____ Power _____

Interval 1:	TIME _____	HR _____	P _____
Interval 2:	TIME _____	HR _____	P _____
Interval 3:	TIME _____	HR _____	P _____
Interval 4:	TIME _____	HR _____	P _____
Interval 5:	TIME _____	HR _____	P _____

Workout Notes _____

Personal Notes _____

Friday ■ Date: ___ / ___ / ___

Waking Heart Rate _____

Standing Heart Rate _____

Waking Weight _____ Hours of Sleep _____

Quality of Sleep 1 2 3 4 5 6 7 8 9 10

Mood State 1 2 3 4 5 6 7 8 9 10

Goal _____

Workout _____

Specific Task _____

Actual Workout Time _____

Distance _____ Cadence _____

Average Heart Rate _____ Power _____

Interval 1:	TIME _____	HR _____	P _____
Interval 2:	TIME _____	HR _____	P _____
Interval 3:	TIME _____	HR _____	P _____
Interval 4:	TIME _____	HR _____	P _____
Interval 5:	TIME _____	HR _____	P _____

Workout Notes _____

Personal Notes _____

Saturday ■ Date: ___ / ___ / ___

Waking Heart Rate _____

Standing Heart Rate _____

Waking Weight _____ Hours of Sleep _____

Quality of Sleep 1 2 3 4 5 6 7 8 9 10

Mood State 1 2 3 4 5 6 7 8 9 10

Goal _____

Workout _____

Specific Task _____

Actual Workout Time _____

Distance _____ Cadence _____

Average Heart Rate _____ Power _____

Interval 1:	TIME _____	HR _____	P _____
Interval 2:	TIME _____	HR _____	P _____
Interval 3:	TIME _____	HR _____	P _____
Interval 4:	TIME _____	HR _____	P _____
Interval 5:	TIME _____	HR _____	P _____

Workout Notes _____

Personal Notes _____

Week #

Sunday ■ Date: ___ / ___ / ___

Waking Heart Rate ___

Standing Heart Rate ___

Waking Weight ___ Hours of Sleep ___

Quality of Sleep 1 2 3 4 5 6 7 8 9 10

Mood State 1 2 3 4 5 6 7 8 9 10

Goal ___

Workout ___

Specific Task ___

Actual Workout Time ___

Distance ___ Cadence ___

Average Heart Rate ___ Power ___

Interval 1: TIME ___ HR ___ P ___
Interval 2: TIME ___ HR ___ P ___
Interval 3: TIME ___ HR ___ P ___
Interval 4: TIME ___ HR ___ P ___
Interval 5: TIME ___ HR ___ P ___

Workout Notes ___

Personal Notes ___

Weekly Summary

Hours of Cycling: ___ Year-to-Date: ___

Miles/Kilometers: ___ Year-to-Date: ___

Hours of Strength Training: ___ Year-to-Date: ___

Hours of Other Activities: ___ Year-to-Date: ___

___ Year-to-Date: ___

___ Year-to-Date: ___

___ Year-to-Date: ___

Total Training Hours: ___

Number of Workouts Planned: ___

Number of Workouts Completed: ___

Average Hours of Sleep: ___

Average Quality of Sleep: ___

Average Mood State: ___

Time Spent in Heart Rate/Power Ranges:

CTS RANGES	TIME	CTS RANGES	TIME	OTHER WORKOUTS	TIME
RecoveryMiles™	___	SteadyState™	___	___	___
FoundationMiles™	___	ClimbingRepeats™	___	___	___
EnduranceMiles™	___	Max Effort	___	___	___
Tempo™	___				

Personal Notes: ___

Weekly Strength Training Record

Exercise	Date:						Date:						Date:					
	SET 1		SET 2		SET 3		SET 1		SET 2		SET 3		SET 1		SET 2		SET 3	
	lbs.	reps	lbs.	reps	lbs.	reps	lbs.	reps	lbs.	reps	lbs.	reps	lbs.	reps	lbs.	reps	lbs.	reps

Race Results

Race #1 _____ Date: ___ / ___ / ___

Time _____ Distance _____

Goal _____

Result _____

Average Heart Rate _____ Power _____

Food/Fluid Intake _____

Personal Notes _____

_____

_____

Race #2 _____ Date: ___ / ___ / ___

Time _____ Distance _____

Goal _____

Result _____

Average Heart Rate _____ Power _____

Food/Fluid Intake _____

Personal Notes _____

_____

_____

Week # _____ Goal: _____

Monday ■ Date: ___ / ___ / ___

Waking Heart Rate _____

Standing Heart Rate _____

Waking Weight _____ Hours of Sleep _____

Quality of Sleep 1 2 3 4 5 6 7 8 9 10

Mood State 1 2 3 4 5 6 7 8 9 10

Goal _____

Workout _____

Specific Task _____

Actual Workout Time _____

Distance _____ Cadence _____

Average Heart Rate _____ Power _____

Interval 1: TIME _____ HR _____ P _____
Interval 2: TIME _____ HR _____ P _____
Interval 3: TIME _____ HR _____ P _____
Interval 4: TIME _____ HR _____ P _____
Interval 5: TIME _____ HR _____ P _____

Workout Notes _____

Personal Notes _____

Tuesday ■ Date: ___ / ___ / ___

Waking Heart Rate _____

Standing Heart Rate _____

Waking Weight _____ Hours of Sleep _____

Quality of Sleep 1 2 3 4 5 6 7 8 9 10

Mood State 1 2 3 4 5 6 7 8 9 10

Goal _____

Workout _____

Specific Task _____

Actual Workout Time _____

Distance _____ Cadence _____

Average Heart Rate _____ Power _____

Interval 1: TIME _____ HR _____ P _____
Interval 2: TIME _____ HR _____ P _____
Interval 3: TIME _____ HR _____ P _____
Interval 4: TIME _____ HR _____ P _____
Interval 5: TIME _____ HR _____ P _____

Workout Notes _____

Personal Notes _____

Wednesday ■ Date: ___ / ___ / ___

Waking Heart Rate _____

Standing Heart Rate _____

Waking Weight _____ Hours of Sleep _____

Quality of Sleep 1 2 3 4 5 6 7 8 9 10

Mood State 1 2 3 4 5 6 7 8 9 10

Goal _____

Workout _____

Specific Task _____

Actual Workout Time _____

Distance _____ Cadence _____

Average Heart Rate _____ Power _____

Interval 1: TIME _____ HR _____ P _____
Interval 2: TIME _____ HR _____ P _____
Interval 3: TIME _____ HR _____ P _____
Interval 4: TIME _____ HR _____ P _____
Interval 5: TIME _____ HR _____ P _____

Workout Notes _____

Personal Notes _____

Thursday ▪ Date: ___/___/___

Waking Heart Rate _____

Standing Heart Rate _____

Waking Weight _____ Hours of Sleep _____

Quality of Sleep 1 2 3 4 5 6 7 8 9 10

Mood State 1 2 3 4 5 6 7 8 9 10

Goal _____

Workout _____

Specific Task _____

Actual Workout Time _____

Distance _____ Cadence _____

Average Heart Rate _____ Power _____

Interval 1: TIME _____ HR _____ P _____

Interval 2: TIME _____ HR _____ P _____

Interval 3: TIME _____ HR _____ P _____

Interval 4: TIME _____ HR _____ P _____

Interval 5: TIME _____ HR _____ P _____

Workout Notes _____

Personal Notes _____

_____

_____

_____

Friday ▪ Date: ___/___/___

Waking Heart Rate _____

Standing Heart Rate _____

Waking Weight _____ Hours of Sleep _____

Quality of Sleep 1 2 3 4 5 6 7 8 9 10

Mood State 1 2 3 4 5 6 7 8 9 10

Goal _____

Workout _____

Specific Task _____

Actual Workout Time _____

Distance _____ Cadence _____

Average Heart Rate _____ Power _____

Interval 1: TIME _____ HR _____ P _____

Interval 2: TIME _____ HR _____ P _____

Interval 3: TIME _____ HR _____ P _____

Interval 4: TIME _____ HR _____ P _____

Interval 5: TIME _____ HR _____ P _____

Workout Notes _____

Personal Notes _____

Saturday ▪ Date: ___/___/___

Waking Heart Rate _____

Standing Heart Rate _____

Waking Weight _____ Hours of Sleep _____

Quality of Sleep 1 2 3 4 5 6 7 8 9 10

Mood State 1 2 3 4 5 6 7 8 9 10

Goal _____

Workout _____

Specific Task _____

Actual Workout Time _____

Distance _____ Cadence _____

Average Heart Rate _____ Power _____

Interval 1: TIME _____ HR _____ P _____

Interval 2: TIME _____ HR _____ P _____

Interval 3: TIME _____ HR _____ P _____

Interval 4: TIME _____ HR _____ P _____

Interval 5: TIME _____ HR _____ P _____

Workout Notes _____

Personal Notes _____

Week # _____

Sunday ■ Date: ____ / ____ / ____

Waking Heart Rate _____

Standing Heart Rate _____

Waking Weight _____ Hours of Sleep _____

Quality of Sleep   1 2 3 4 5 6 7 8 9 10

Mood State   1 2 3 4 5 6 7 8 9 10

Goal _____

Workout _____

Specific Task _____

Actual Workout Time _____

Distance _____ Cadence _____

Average Heart Rate _____ Power _____

Interval 1: TIME _____ HR _____ P _____

Interval 2: TIME _____ HR _____ P _____

Interval 3: TIME _____ HR _____ P _____

Interval 4: TIME _____ HR _____ P _____

Interval 5: TIME _____ HR _____ P _____

Workout Notes _____

Personal Notes _____

Weekly Summary

Hours of Cycling: _____ Year-to-Date: _____

Miles/Kilometers: _____ Year-to-Date: _____

Hours of Strength Training: _____ Year-to-Date: _____

Hours of Other Activities: _____ Year-to-Date: _____

_____ Year-to-Date: _____

_____ Year-to-Date: _____

Total Training Hours: _____ Year-to-Date: _____

Number of Workouts Planned: _____

Number of Workouts Completed: _____

Average Hours of Sleep: _____

Average Quality of Sleep: _____

Average Mood State: _____

Time Spent in Heart Rate/Power Ranges:

CTS RANGES	TIME	CTS RANGES	TIME	OTHER WORKOUTS	TIME
RecoveryMiles™		SteadyState™			
FoundationMiles™		ClimbingRepeats™			
EnduranceMiles™		Max Effort			
Tempo™					

Personal Notes: _____

Week #___ Weekly Strength Training Record

Exercise	Date:								
	SET 1 lbs. / reps	**SET 2** lbs. / reps	**SET 3** lbs. / reps	**SET 1** lbs. / reps	**SET 2** lbs. / reps	**SET 3** lbs. / reps	**SET 1** lbs. / reps	**SET 2** lbs. / reps	**SET 3** lbs. / reps

(Date: ___ columns repeated across the top)

Race Results

Race #1_____ Date: ___/___/___

Time_____ Distance_____

Goal_____

Result_____

Average Heart Rate_____ Power_____

Food/Fluid Intake_____

Personal Notes_____

_____

_____

Race #2_____ Date: ___/___/___

Time_____ Distance_____

Goal_____

Result_____

Average Heart Rate_____ Power_____

Food/Fluid Intake_____

Personal Notes_____

_____

_____

Week #   Goal: _____

Monday ■ Date: ___ / ___ / ___

Waking Heart Rate _____

Standing Heart Rate _____

Waking Weight _____ Hours of Sleep _____

Quality of Sleep 1 2 3 4 5 6 7 8 9 10

Mood State 1 2 3 4 5 6 7 8 9 10

Goal _____

Workout _____

Specific Task _____

Actual Workout Time _____

Distance _____ Cadence _____ Power _____

Average Heart Rate _____ Power _____

Interval 1: TIME ____ HR ____ P ____
Interval 2: TIME ____ HR ____ P ____
Interval 3: TIME ____ HR ____ P ____
Interval 4: TIME ____ HR ____ P ____
Interval 5: TIME ____ HR ____ P ____

Workout Notes _____

Personal Notes _____

Tuesday ■ Date: ___ / ___ / ___

Waking Heart Rate _____

Standing Heart Rate _____

Waking Weight _____ Hours of Sleep _____

Quality of Sleep 1 2 3 4 5 6 7 8 9 10

Mood State 1 2 3 4 5 6 7 8 9 10

Goal _____

Workout _____

Specific Task _____

Actual Workout Time _____

Distance _____ Cadence _____ Power _____

Average Heart Rate _____ Power _____

Interval 1: TIME ____ HR ____ P ____
Interval 2: TIME ____ HR ____ P ____
Interval 3: TIME ____ HR ____ P ____
Interval 4: TIME ____ HR ____ P ____
Interval 5: TIME ____ HR ____ P ____

Workout Notes _____

Personal Notes _____

Wednesday ■ Date: ___ / ___ / ___

Waking Heart Rate _____

Standing Heart Rate _____

Waking Weight _____ Hours of Sleep _____

Quality of Sleep 1 2 3 4 5 6 7 8 9 10

Mood State 1 2 3 4 5 6 7 8 9 10

Goal _____

Workout _____

Specific Task _____

Actual Workout Time _____

Distance _____ Cadence _____ Power _____

Average Heart Rate _____ Power _____

Interval 1: TIME ____ HR ____ P ____
Interval 2: TIME ____ HR ____ P ____
Interval 3: TIME ____ HR ____ P ____
Interval 4: TIME ____ HR ____ P ____
Interval 5: TIME ____ HR ____ P ____

Workout Notes _____

Personal Notes _____

Thursday ▪ Date: ___ / ___ / ___

Waking Heart Rate _____

Standing Heart Rate _____

Waking Weight _____ Hours of Sleep _____

Quality of Sleep 1 2 3 4 5 6 7 8 9 10

Mood State 1 2 3 4 5 6 7 8 9 10

Goal _____

Workout _____

Specific Task _____

Actual Workout Time _____

Distance _____ Cadence _____ Power _____

Average Heart Rate _____

Interval 1:	TIME ___	HR ___	P ___
Interval 2:	TIME ___	HR ___	P ___
Interval 3:	TIME ___	HR ___	P ___
Interval 4:	TIME ___	HR ___	P ___
Interval 5:	TIME ___	HR ___	P ___

Workout Notes _____

Personal Notes _____

Friday ▪ Date: ___ / ___ / ___

Waking Heart Rate _____

Standing Heart Rate _____

Waking Weight _____ Hours of Sleep _____

Quality of Sleep 1 2 3 4 5 6 7 8 9 10

Mood State 1 2 3 4 5 6 7 8 9 10

Goal _____

Workout _____

Specific Task _____

Actual Workout Time _____

Distance _____ Cadence _____ Power _____

Average Heart Rate _____

Interval 1:	TIME ___	HR ___	P ___
Interval 2:	TIME ___	HR ___	P ___
Interval 3:	TIME ___	HR ___	P ___
Interval 4:	TIME ___	HR ___	P ___
Interval 5:	TIME ___	HR ___	P ___

Workout Notes _____

Personal Notes _____

Saturday ▪ Date: ___ / ___ / ___

Waking Heart Rate _____

Standing Heart Rate _____

Waking Weight _____ Hours of Sleep _____

Quality of Sleep 1 2 3 4 5 6 7 8 9 10

Mood State 1 2 3 4 5 6 7 8 9 10

Goal _____

Workout _____

Specific Task _____

Actual Workout Time _____

Distance _____ Cadence _____ Power _____

Average Heart Rate _____

Interval 1:	TIME ___	HR ___	P ___
Interval 2:	TIME ___	HR ___	P ___
Interval 3:	TIME ___	HR ___	P ___
Interval 4:	TIME ___	HR ___	P ___
Interval 5:	TIME ___	HR ___	P ___

Workout Notes _____

Personal Notes _____

Week #

Sunday ■ Date: ___/___/___

Waking Heart Rate _____

Standing Heart Rate _____

Waking Weight _____ Hours of Sleep _____

Quality of Sleep   1 2 3 4 5 6 7 8 9 10

Mood State   1 2 3 4 5 6 7 8 9 10

Goal _____

Workout _____

Specific Task _____

Actual Workout Time _____

Distance _____ Cadence _____

Average Heart Rate _____ Power _____

Interval 1:	TIME _____	HR _____	P _____
Interval 2:	TIME _____	HR _____	P _____
Interval 3:	TIME _____	HR _____	P _____
Interval 4:	TIME _____	HR _____	P _____
Interval 5:	TIME _____	HR _____	P _____

Workout Notes _____

Personal Notes _____

Weekly Summary

Hours of Cycling: _____ Year-to-Date: _____

Miles/Kilometers: _____ Year-to-Date: _____

Hours of Strength Training: _____ Year-to-Date: _____

Hours of Other Activities: _____

_____ Year-to-Date: _____

_____ Year-to-Date: _____

Total Training Hours: _____ Year-to-Date: _____

Number of Workouts Planned: _____

Number of Workouts Completed: _____

Average Hours of Sleep: _____

Average Quality of Sleep: _____

Average Mood State: _____

Time Spent in Heart Rate/Power Ranges:

CTS RANGES	TIME	CTS RANGES	TIME	OTHER WORKOUTS	TIME
RecoveryMiles™		SteadyState™			
FoundationMiles™		ClimbingRepeats™			
EnduranceMiles™		Max Effort			
Tempo™					

Personal Notes: _____

Weekly Strength Training Record

Race Results

Exercise	Date:						Date:						Date:					
	SET 1		SET 2		SET 3		SET 1		SET 2		SET 3		SET 1		SET 2		SET 3	
	lbs.	reps	lbs.	reps	lbs.	reps	lbs.	reps	lbs.	reps	lbs.	reps	lbs.	reps	lbs.	reps	lbs.	reps

Race #1 _____ Date: ___ / ___ / ___

Time _____ Distance _____

Goal _____

Result _____

Average Heart Rate _____ Power _____

Food/Fluid Intake _____

Personal Notes _____

_____

Race #2 _____ Date: ___ / ___ / ___

Time _____ Distance _____

Goal _____

Result _____

Average Heart Rate _____ Power _____

Food/Fluid Intake _____

Personal Notes _____

_____

Week # _____   Goal: _____

Monday ■ Date: ___ / ___ / ___

Waking Heart Rate _____
Standing Heart Rate _____
Waking Weight _____ Hours of Sleep _____
Quality of Sleep 1 2 3 4 5 6 7 8 9 10

Mood State 1 2 3 4 5 6 7 8 9 10

Goal _____
Workout _____
Specific Task _____
Actual Workout Time _____
Distance _____ Cadence _____
Average Heart Rate _____ Power _____

Interval 1: TIME _____ HR _____ P _____
Interval 2: TIME _____ HR _____ P _____
Interval 3: TIME _____ HR _____ P _____
Interval 4: TIME _____ HR _____ P _____
Interval 5: TIME _____ HR _____ P _____

Workout Notes _____

Personal Notes _____

Tuesday ■ Date: ___ / ___ / ___

Waking Heart Rate _____
Standing Heart Rate _____
Waking Weight _____ Hours of Sleep _____
Quality of Sleep 1 2 3 4 5 6 7 8 9 10

Mood State 1 2 3 4 5 6 7 8 9 10

Goal _____
Workout _____
Specific Task _____
Actual Workout Time _____
Distance _____ Cadence _____
Average Heart Rate _____ Power _____

Interval 1: TIME _____ HR _____ P _____
Interval 2: TIME _____ HR _____ P _____
Interval 3: TIME _____ HR _____ P _____
Interval 4: TIME _____ HR _____ P _____
Interval 5: TIME _____ HR _____ P _____

Workout Notes _____

Personal Notes _____

Wednesday ■ Date: ___ / ___ / ___

Waking Heart Rate _____
Standing Heart Rate _____
Waking Weight _____ Hours of Sleep _____
Quality of Sleep 1 2 3 4 5 6 7 8 9 10

Mood State 1 2 3 4 5 6 7 8 9 10

Goal _____
Workout _____
Specific Task _____
Actual Workout Time _____
Distance _____ Cadence _____
Average Heart Rate _____ Power _____

Interval 1: TIME _____ HR _____ P _____
Interval 2: TIME _____ HR _____ P _____
Interval 3: TIME _____ HR _____ P _____
Interval 4: TIME _____ HR _____ P _____
Interval 5: TIME _____ HR _____ P _____

Workout Notes _____

Personal Notes _____

Thursday ■ Date: ___ / ___ / ___

Waking Heart Rate ___

Standing Heart Rate ___

Waking Weight ___ Hours of Sleep ___

Quality of Sleep 1 2 3 4 5 6 7 8 9 10

Mood State 1 2 3 4 5 6 7 8 9 10

Goal ___

Workout ___

Specific Task ___

Actual Workout Time ___

Distance ___ Cadence ___

Average Heart Rate ___ Power ___

Interval 1: TIME ___ HR ___ P ___
Interval 2: TIME ___ HR ___ P ___
Interval 3: TIME ___ HR ___ P ___
Interval 4: TIME ___ HR ___ P ___
Interval 5: TIME ___ HR ___ P ___

Workout Notes ___

Personal Notes ___

Friday ■ Date: ___ / ___ / ___

Waking Heart Rate ___

Standing Heart Rate ___

Waking Weight ___ Hours of Sleep ___

Quality of Sleep 1 2 3 4 5 6 7 8 9 10

Mood State 1 2 3 4 5 6 7 8 9 10

Goal ___

Workout ___

Specific Task ___

Actual Workout Time ___

Distance ___ Cadence ___

Average Heart Rate ___ Power ___

Interval 1: TIME ___ HR ___ P ___
Interval 2: TIME ___ HR ___ P ___
Interval 3: TIME ___ HR ___ P ___
Interval 4: TIME ___ HR ___ P ___
Interval 5: TIME ___ HR ___ P ___

Workout Notes ___

Personal Notes ___

Saturday ■ Date: ___ / ___ / ___

Waking Heart Rate ___

Standing Heart Rate ___

Waking Weight ___ Hours of Sleep ___

Quality of Sleep 1 2 3 4 5 6 7 8 9 10

Mood State 1 2 3 4 5 6 7 8 9 10

Goal ___

Workout ___

Specific Task ___

Actual Workout Time ___

Distance ___ Cadence ___

Average Heart Rate ___ Power ___

Interval 1: TIME ___ HR ___ P ___
Interval 2: TIME ___ HR ___ P ___
Interval 3: TIME ___ HR ___ P ___
Interval 4: TIME ___ HR ___ P ___
Interval 5: TIME ___ HR ___ P ___

Workout Notes ___

Personal Notes ___

Week #

Sunday ■ Date: ___ / ___ / ___

Waking Heart Rate _____

Standing Heart Rate _____

Waking Weight _____ Hours of Sleep _____

Quality of Sleep 1 2 3 4 5 6 7 8 9 10

Mood State 1 2 3 4 5 6 7 8 9 10

Goal _____

Workout _____

Specific Task _____

Actual Workout Time _____

Distance _____ Cadence _____

Average Heart Rate _____ Power _____

Interval 1: TIME _____ HR _____ P _____
Interval 2: TIME _____ HR _____ P _____
Interval 3: TIME _____ HR _____ P _____
Interval 4: TIME _____ HR _____ P _____
Interval 5: TIME _____ HR _____ P _____

Workout Notes _____

Personal Notes _____

Weekly Summary

Hours of Cycling: _____ Year-to-Date: _____

Miles/Kilometers: _____ Year-to-Date: _____

Hours of Strength Training: _____ Year-to-Date: _____

Hours of Other Activities: _____ Year-to-Date: _____

_____ Year-to-Date: _____

_____ Year-to-Date: _____

_____ Year-to-Date: _____

Total Training Hours: _____

Number of Workouts Planned: _____

Number of Workouts Completed: _____

Average Hours of Sleep: _____

Average Quality of Sleep: _____

Average Mood State: _____

Time Spent in Heart Rate/Power Ranges:

CTS RANGES	TIME	CTS RANGES	TIME	OTHER WORKOUTS	TIME
RecoveryMiles™		SteadyState™			
FoundationMiles™		ClimbingRepeats™			
EnduranceMiles™		Max Effort			
Tempo™					

Personal Notes: _____

Race Results

Race #1 _____ Date: ___/___/___

Time_____ Distance_____

Goal_____

Result_____

Average Heart Rate_____ Power_____

Food/Fluid Intake_____

Personal Notes_____

Race #2 _____ Date: ___/___/___

Time_____ Distance_____

Goal_____

Result_____

Average Heart Rate_____ Power_____

Food/Fluid Intake_____

Personal Notes_____

Week # _____

Weekly Strength Training Record

Exercise	Date:			Date:			Date:		
	SET 1 lbs./reps	SET 2 lbs./reps	SET 3 lbs./reps	SET 1 lbs./reps	SET 2 lbs./reps	SET 3 lbs./reps	SET 1 lbs./reps	SET 2 lbs./reps	SET 3 lbs./reps

Week # _____   **Goal:** _____

Monday ■ Date: ___ / ___ / ___

Waking Heart Rate _____

Standing Heart Rate _____

Waking Weight _____ Hours of Sleep _____

Quality of Sleep   1 2 3 4 5 6 7 8 9 10

Mood State   1 2 3 4 5 6 7 8 9 10

Goal _____

Workout _____

Specific Task _____

Actual Workout Time _____

Distance _____ Cadence _____ Power _____

Average Heart Rate _____

Interval 1: TIME _____ HR _____ P _____
Interval 2: TIME _____ HR _____ P _____
Interval 3: TIME _____ HR _____ P _____
Interval 4: TIME _____ HR _____ P _____
Interval 5: TIME _____ HR _____ P _____

Workout Notes _____

Personal Notes _____

Tuesday ■ Date: ___ / ___ / ___

Waking Heart Rate _____

Standing Heart Rate _____

Waking Weight _____ Hours of Sleep _____

Quality of Sleep   1 2 3 4 5 6 7 8 9 10

Mood State   1 2 3 4 5 6 7 8 9 10

Goal _____

Workout _____

Specific Task _____

Actual Workout Time _____

Distance _____ Cadence _____ Power _____

Average Heart Rate _____

Interval 1: TIME _____ HR _____ P _____
Interval 2: TIME _____ HR _____ P _____
Interval 3: TIME _____ HR _____ P _____
Interval 4: TIME _____ HR _____ P _____
Interval 5: TIME _____ HR _____ P _____

Workout Notes _____

Personal Notes _____

Wednesday ■ Date: ___ / ___ / ___

Waking Heart Rate _____

Standing Heart Rate _____

Waking Weight _____ Hours of Sleep _____

Quality of Sleep   1 2 3 4 5 6 7 8 9 10

Mood State   1 2 3 4 5 6 7 8 9 10

Goal _____

Workout _____

Specific Task _____

Actual Workout Time _____

Distance _____ Cadence _____ Power _____

Average Heart Rate _____

Interval 1: TIME _____ HR _____ P _____
Interval 2: TIME _____ HR _____ P _____
Interval 3: TIME _____ HR _____ P _____
Interval 4: TIME _____ HR _____ P _____
Interval 5: TIME _____ HR _____ P _____

Workout Notes _____

Personal Notes _____

Thursday ■ Date: ___ / ___ / ___

Waking Heart Rate ___

Standing Heart Rate ___

Waking Weight ___ Hours of Sleep ___

Quality of Sleep 1 2 3 4 5 6 7 8 9 10

Mood State 1 2 3 4 5 6 7 8 9 10

Goal ___

Workout ___

Specific Task ___

Actual Workout Time ___

Distance ___ Cadence ___

Average Heart Rate ___ Power ___

Interval 1: TIME ___ HR ___ P ___

Interval 2: TIME ___ HR ___ P ___

Interval 3: TIME ___ HR ___ P ___

Interval 4: TIME ___ HR ___ P ___

Interval 5: TIME ___ HR ___ P ___

Workout Notes ___

Personal Notes ___

Friday ■ Date: ___ / ___ / ___

Waking Heart Rate ___

Standing Heart Rate ___

Waking Weight ___ Hours of Sleep ___

Quality of Sleep 1 2 3 4 5 6 7 8 9 10

Mood State 1 2 3 4 5 6 7 8 9 10

Goal ___

Workout ___

Specific Task ___

Actual Workout Time ___

Distance ___ Cadence ___

Average Heart Rate ___ Power ___

Interval 1: TIME ___ HR ___ P ___

Interval 2: TIME ___ HR ___ P ___

Interval 3: TIME ___ HR ___ P ___

Interval 4: TIME ___ HR ___ P ___

Interval 5: TIME ___ HR ___ P ___

Workout Notes ___

Personal Notes ___

Saturday ■ Date: ___ / ___ / ___

Waking Heart Rate ___

Standing Heart Rate ___

Waking Weight ___ Hours of Sleep ___

Quality of Sleep 1 2 3 4 5 6 7 8 9 10

Mood State 1 2 3 4 5 6 7 8 9 10

Goal ___

Workout ___

Specific Task ___

Actual Workout Time ___

Distance ___ Cadence ___

Average Heart Rate ___ Power ___

Interval 1: TIME ___ HR ___ P ___

Interval 2: TIME ___ HR ___ P ___

Interval 3: TIME ___ HR ___ P ___

Interval 4: TIME ___ HR ___ P ___

Interval 5: TIME ___ HR ___ P ___

Workout Notes ___

Personal Notes ___

Sunday ■ Date: ___ / ___ / ___

Waking Heart Rate _____

Standing Heart Rate _____

Waking Weight _____ Hours of Sleep _____

Quality of Sleep 1 2 3 4 5 6 7 8 9 10

Mood State 1 2 3 4 5 6 7 8 9 10

Goal _____

Workout _____

Specific Task _____

Actual Workout Time _____

Distance _____ Cadence _____

Average Heart Rate _____ Power _____

Interval 1:	TIME _____	HR _____	P _____
Interval 2:	TIME _____	HR _____	P _____
Interval 3:	TIME _____	HR _____	P _____
Interval 4:	TIME _____	HR _____	P _____
Interval 5:	TIME _____	HR _____	P _____

Workout Notes _____

Personal Notes _____

Weekly Summary

Hours of Cycling: _____ Year-to-Date: _____

Miles/Kilometers: _____ Year-to-Date: _____

Hours of Strength Training: _____ Year-to-Date: _____

Hours of Other Activities: _____

_____ Year-to-Date: _____

_____ Year-to-Date: _____

_____ Year-to-Date: _____

_____ Year-to-Date: _____

Total Training Hours: _____

Number of Workouts Planned: _____

Number of Workouts Completed: _____

Average Hours of Sleep: _____

Average Quality of Sleep: _____

Average Mood State: _____

Time Spent in Heart Rate/Power Ranges:

CTS RANGES	TIME	CTS RANGES	TIME	OTHER WORKOUTS	TIME
RecoveryMiles™		SteadyState™			
FoundationMiles™		ClimbingRepeats™			
EnduranceMiles™		Max Effort			
Tempo™					

Personal Notes: _____

Weekly Strength Training Record

Exercise	Date:			Date:			Date:		
	SET 1 lbs. / reps	SET 2 lbs. / reps	SET 3 lbs. / reps	SET 1 lbs. / reps	SET 2 lbs. / reps	SET 3 lbs. / reps	SET 1 lbs. / reps	SET 2 lbs. / reps	SET 3 lbs. / reps

Race Results

Race #1 _____ Date: ___/___/___

Time _____ Distance _____

Goal _____

Result _____

Average Heart Rate _____ Power _____

Food/Fluid Intake _____

Personal Notes _____

_____

_____

Race #2 _____ Date: ___/___/___

Time _____ Distance _____

Goal _____

Result _____

Average Heart Rate _____ Power _____

Food/Fluid Intake _____

Personal Notes _____

_____

_____

Week # _____   Goal: _____

Monday ■ Date: ____ / ____ / ____

Waking Heart Rate _____

Standing Heart Rate _____

Waking Weight _____ Hours of Sleep _____

Quality of Sleep 1 2 3 4 5 6 7 8 9 10

Mood State 1 2 3 4 5 6 7 8 9 10

Goal _____

Workout _____

Specific Task _____

Actual Workout Time _____

Distance _____ Cadence _____

Average Heart Rate _____ Power _____

Interval 1: TIME _____ HR _____ P _____
Interval 2: TIME _____ HR _____ P _____
Interval 3: TIME _____ HR _____ P _____
Interval 4: TIME _____ HR _____ P _____
Interval 5: TIME _____ HR _____ P _____

Workout Notes _____

Personal Notes _____

Tuesday ■ Date: ____ / ____ / ____

Waking Heart Rate _____

Standing Heart Rate _____

Waking Weight _____ Hours of Sleep _____

Quality of Sleep 1 2 3 4 5 6 7 8 9 10

Mood State 1 2 3 4 5 6 7 8 9 10

Goal _____

Workout _____

Specific Task _____

Actual Workout Time _____

Distance _____ Cadence _____

Average Heart Rate _____ Power _____

Interval 1: TIME _____ HR _____ P _____
Interval 2: TIME _____ HR _____ P _____
Interval 3: TIME _____ HR _____ P _____
Interval 4: TIME _____ HR _____ P _____
Interval 5: TIME _____ HR _____ P _____

Workout Notes _____

Personal Notes _____

Wednesday ■ Date: ____ / ____ / ____

Waking Heart Rate _____

Standing Heart Rate _____

Waking Weight _____ Hours of Sleep _____

Quality of Sleep 1 2 3 4 5 6 7 8 9 10

Mood State 1 2 3 4 5 6 7 8 9 10

Goal _____

Workout _____

Specific Task _____

Actual Workout Time _____

Distance _____ Cadence _____

Average Heart Rate _____ Power _____

Interval 1: TIME _____ HR _____ P _____
Interval 2: TIME _____ HR _____ P _____
Interval 3: TIME _____ HR _____ P _____
Interval 4: TIME _____ HR _____ P _____
Interval 5: TIME _____ HR _____ P _____

Workout Notes _____

Personal Notes _____

Thursday ■ Date: ___ / ___ / ___

Waking Heart Rate ___

Standing Heart Rate ___

Waking Weight ___ Hours of Sleep ___

Quality of Sleep 1 2 3 4 5 6 7 8 9 10

Mood State 1 2 3 4 5 6 7 8 9 10

Goal ___

Workout ___

Specific Task ___

Actual Workout Time ___

Distance ___ Cadence ___

Average Heart Rate ___ Power ___

Interval 1: TIME ___ HR ___ P ___

Interval 2: TIME ___ HR ___ P ___

Interval 3: TIME ___ HR ___ P ___

Interval 4: TIME ___ HR ___ P ___

Interval 5: TIME ___ HR ___ P ___

Workout Notes ___

Personal Notes ___

Friday ■ Date: ___ / ___ / ___

Waking Heart Rate ___

Standing Heart Rate ___

Waking Weight ___ Hours of Sleep ___

Quality of Sleep 1 2 3 4 5 6 7 8 9 10

Mood State 1 2 3 4 5 6 7 8 9 10

Goal ___

Workout ___

Specific Task ___

Actual Workout Time ___

Distance ___ Cadence ___

Average Heart Rate ___ Power ___

Interval 1: TIME ___ HR ___ P ___

Interval 2: TIME ___ HR ___ P ___

Interval 3: TIME ___ HR ___ P ___

Interval 4: TIME ___ HR ___ P ___

Interval 5: TIME ___ HR ___ P ___

Workout Notes ___

Personal Notes ___

Saturday ■ Date: ___ / ___ / ___

Waking Heart Rate ___

Standing Heart Rate ___

Waking Weight ___ Hours of Sleep ___

Quality of Sleep 1 2 3 4 5 6 7 8 9 10

Mood State 1 2 3 4 5 6 7 8 9 10

Goal ___

Workout ___

Specific Task ___

Actual Workout Time ___

Distance ___ Cadence ___

Average Heart Rate ___ Power ___

Interval 1: TIME ___ HR ___ P ___

Interval 2: TIME ___ HR ___ P ___

Interval 3: TIME ___ HR ___ P ___

Interval 4: TIME ___ HR ___ P ___

Interval 5: TIME ___ HR ___ P ___

Workout Notes ___

Personal Notes ___

Sunday ■ Date: _____ / _____ / _____

Waking Heart Rate _____

Standing Heart Rate _____

Waking Weight _____ Hours of Sleep _____

Quality of Sleep 1 2 3 4 5 6 7 8 9 10

Mood State 1 2 3 4 5 6 7 8 9 10

Goal _____

Workout _____

Specific Task _____

Actual Workout Time _____

Distance _____ Cadence _____

Average Heart Rate _____ Power _____

Interval 1: TIME _____ HR _____ P _____

Interval 2: TIME _____ HR _____ P _____

Interval 3: TIME _____ HR _____ P _____

Interval 4: TIME _____ HR _____ P _____

Interval 5: TIME _____ HR _____ P _____

Workout Notes _____

Personal Notes _____

Weekly Summary

Hours of Cycling: _____ Year-to-Date: _____

Miles/Kilometers: _____ Year-to-Date: _____

Hours of Strength Training: _____ Year-to-Date: _____

Hours of Other Activities: _____

_____ Year-to-Date: _____

_____ Year-to-Date: _____

_____ Year-to-Date: _____

_____ Year-to-Date: _____

Total Training Hours: _____

Number of Workouts Planned: _____

Number of Workouts Completed: _____

Average Hours of Sleep: _____

Average Quality of Sleep: _____

Average Mood State: _____

Time Spent in Heart Rate/Power Ranges:

CTS RANGES	TIME	CTS RANGES	TIME	OTHER WORKOUTS	TIME
RecoveryMiles™		SteadyState™			
FoundationMiles™		ClimbingRepeats™			
EnduranceMiles™		Max Effort			
Tempo™					

Personal Notes: _____

Race Results

Race #1 _____ Date: ___/___/___

Time _____ Distance _____

Goal _____

Result _____

Average Heart Rate _____ Power _____

Food/Fluid Intake _____

Personal Notes _____

_____

_____

Race #2 _____ Date: ___/___/___

Time _____ Distance _____

Goal _____

Result _____

Average Heart Rate _____ Power _____

Food/Fluid Intake _____

Personal Notes _____

_____

_____

Week # _____

Weekly Strength Training Record

Exercise	Date:						Date:						Date:					
	SET 1		SET 2		SET 3		SET 1		SET 2		SET 3		SET 1		SET 2		SET 3	
	lbs.	reps	lbs.	reps	lbs.	reps	lbs.	reps	lbs.	reps	lbs.	reps	lbs.	reps	lbs.	reps	lbs.	reps

Monday ▪ Date: ___ / ___ / ___

Waking Heart Rate _____

Standing Heart Rate _____

Waking Weight _____ Hours of Sleep _____

Quality of Sleep 1 2 3 4 5 6 7 8 9 10

Mood State 1 2 3 4 5 6 7 8 9 10

Goal _____

Workout _____

Specific Task _____

Actual Workout Time _____

Distance _____ Cadence _____

Average Heart Rate _____ Power _____

Interval 1: TIME _____ HR _____ P _____

Interval 2: TIME _____ HR _____ P _____

Interval 3: TIME _____ HR _____ P _____

Interval 4: TIME _____ HR _____ P _____

Interval 5: TIME _____ HR _____ P _____

Workout Notes _____

Personal Notes _____

Tuesday ▪ Date: ___ / ___ / ___

Waking Heart Rate _____

Standing Heart Rate _____

Waking Weight _____ Hours of Sleep _____

Quality of Sleep 1 2 3 4 5 6 7 8 9 10

Mood State 1 2 3 4 5 6 7 8 9 10

Goal _____

Workout _____

Specific Task _____

Actual Workout Time _____

Distance _____ Cadence _____

Average Heart Rate _____ Power _____

Interval 1: TIME _____ HR _____ P _____

Interval 2: TIME _____ HR _____ P _____

Interval 3: TIME _____ HR _____ P _____

Interval 4: TIME _____ HR _____ P _____

Interval 5: TIME _____ HR _____ P _____

Workout Notes _____

Personal Notes _____

Wednesday ▪ Date: ___ / ___ / ___

Waking Heart Rate _____

Standing Heart Rate _____

Waking Weight _____ Hours of Sleep _____

Quality of Sleep 1 2 3 4 5 6 7 8 9 10

Mood State 1 2 3 4 5 6 7 8 9 10

Goal _____

Workout _____

Specific Task _____

Actual Workout Time _____

Distance _____ Cadence _____

Average Heart Rate _____ Power _____

Interval 1: TIME _____ HR _____ P _____

Interval 2: TIME _____ HR _____ P _____

Interval 3: TIME _____ HR _____ P _____

Interval 4: TIME _____ HR _____ P _____

Interval 5: TIME _____ HR _____ P _____

Workout Notes _____

Personal Notes _____

Thursday ■ Date: ___ / ___ / ___

Waking Heart Rate ___

Standing Heart Rate ___

Waking Weight ___ Hours of Sleep ___

Quality of Sleep 1 2 3 4 5 6 7 8 9 10

Mood State 1 2 3 4 5 6 7 8 9 10

Goal ___

Workout ___

Specific Task ___

Actual Workout Time ___

Distance ___ Cadence ___

Average Heart Rate ___ Power ___

Interval 1: TIME ___ HR ___ P ___

Interval 2: TIME ___ HR ___ P ___

Interval 3: TIME ___ HR ___ P ___

Interval 4: TIME ___ HR ___ P ___

Interval 5: TIME ___ HR ___ P ___

Workout Notes ___

Personal Notes ___

Friday ■ Date: ___ / ___ / ___

Waking Heart Rate ___

Standing Heart Rate ___

Waking Weight ___ Hours of Sleep ___

Quality of Sleep 1 2 3 4 5 6 7 8 9 10

Mood State 1 2 3 4 5 6 7 8 9 10

Goal ___

Workout ___

Specific Task ___

Actual Workout Time ___

Distance ___ Cadence ___

Average Heart Rate ___ Power ___

Interval 1: TIME ___ HR ___ P ___

Interval 2: TIME ___ HR ___ P ___

Interval 3: TIME ___ HR ___ P ___

Interval 4: TIME ___ HR ___ P ___

Interval 5: TIME ___ HR ___ P ___

Workout Notes ___

Personal Notes ___

Saturday ■ Date: ___ / ___ / ___

Waking Heart Rate ___

Standing Heart Rate ___

Waking Weight ___ Hours of Sleep ___

Quality of Sleep 1 2 3 4 5 6 7 8 9 10

Mood State 1 2 3 4 5 6 7 8 9 10

Goal ___

Workout ___

Specific Task ___

Actual Workout Time ___

Distance ___ Cadence ___

Average Heart Rate ___ Power ___

Interval 1: TIME ___ HR ___ P ___

Interval 2: TIME ___ HR ___ P ___

Interval 3: TIME ___ HR ___ P ___

Interval 4: TIME ___ HR ___ P ___

Interval 5: TIME ___ HR ___ P ___

Workout Notes ___

Personal Notes ___

Week # _____

Sunday ■ Date: ___ / ___ / ___

Waking Heart Rate _____

Standing Heart Rate _____

Waking Weight _____ Hours of Sleep _____

Quality of Sleep 1 2 3 4 5 6 7 8 9 10

Mood State 1 2 3 4 5 6 7 8 9 10

Goal _____

Workout _____

Specific Task _____

Actual Workout Time _____

Distance _____ Cadence _____

Average Heart Rate _____ Power _____

Interval 1: TIME _____ HR _____ P _____
Interval 2: TIME _____ HR _____ P _____
Interval 3: TIME _____ HR _____ P _____
Interval 4: TIME _____ HR _____ P _____
Interval 5: TIME _____ HR _____ P _____

Workout Notes _____

Personal Notes _____

Weekly Summary

Hours of Cycling: _____ Year-to-Date: _____

Miles/Kilometers: _____ Year-to-Date: _____

Hours of Strength Training: _____ Year-to-Date: _____

Hours of Other Activities: _____

_____ Year-to-Date: _____

_____ Year-to-Date: _____

_____ Year-to-Date: _____

Total Training Hours: _____ Year-to-Date: _____

Number of Workouts Planned: _____

Number of Workouts Completed: _____

Average Hours of Sleep: _____

Average Quality of Sleep: _____

Average Mood State: _____

Time Spent in Heart Rate/Power Ranges:

CTS RANGES	TIME	CTS RANGES	TIME	OTHER WORKOUTS	TIME
RecoveryMiles™		SteadyState™			
FoundationMiles™		ClimbingRepeats™			
EnduranceMiles™		Max Effort			
Tempo™					

Personal Notes: _____

Race Results

Race #1 _____ Date: ___/___/___

Time_____ Distance_____

Goal_____

Result_____

Average Heart Rate_____ Power_____

Food/Fluid Intake_____

Personal Notes_____

_____

_____

Race #2 _____ Date: ___/___/___

Time_____ Distance_____

Goal_____

Result_____

Average Heart Rate_____ Power_____

Food/Fluid Intake_____

Personal Notes_____

_____

_____

Weekly Strength Training Record

Week # _____

Exercise	Date:						Date:						Date:					
	SET 1		SET 2		SET 3		SET 1		SET 2		SET 3		SET 1		SET 2		SET 3	
	lbs.	reps	lbs.	reps	lbs.	reps	lbs.	reps	lbs.	reps	lbs.	reps	lbs.	reps	lbs.	reps	lbs.	reps

Week # _____   Goal: _____

Monday ■ Date: ___ / ___ / ___

Waking Heart Rate _____

Standing Heart Rate _____

Waking Weight _____ Hours of Sleep _____

Quality of Sleep   1 2 3 4 5 6 7 8 9 10

Mood State   1 2 3 4 5 6 7 8 9 10

Goal _____

Workout _____

Specific Task _____

Actual Workout Time _____

Distance _____ Cadence _____

Average Heart Rate _____ Power _____

Interval 1: TIME _____ HR _____ P _____
Interval 2: TIME _____ HR _____ P _____
Interval 3: TIME _____ HR _____ P _____
Interval 4: TIME _____ HR _____ P _____
Interval 5: TIME _____ HR _____ P _____

Workout Notes _____

Personal Notes _____

Tuesday ■ Date: ___ / ___ / ___

Waking Heart Rate _____

Standing Heart Rate _____

Waking Weight _____ Hours of Sleep _____

Quality of Sleep   1 2 3 4 5 6 7 8 9 10

Mood State   1 2 3 4 5 6 7 8 9 10

Goal _____

Workout _____

Specific Task _____

Actual Workout Time _____

Distance _____ Cadence _____

Average Heart Rate _____ Power _____

Interval 1: TIME _____ HR _____ P _____
Interval 2: TIME _____ HR _____ P _____
Interval 3: TIME _____ HR _____ P _____
Interval 4: TIME _____ HR _____ P _____
Interval 5: TIME _____ HR _____ P _____

Workout Notes _____

Personal Notes _____

Wednesday ■ Date: ___ / ___ / ___

Waking Heart Rate _____

Standing Heart Rate _____

Waking Weight _____ Hours of Sleep _____

Quality of Sleep   1 2 3 4 5 6 7 8 9 10

Mood State   1 2 3 4 5 6 7 8 9 10

Goal _____

Workout _____

Specific Task _____

Actual Workout Time _____

Distance _____ Cadence _____

Average Heart Rate _____ Power _____

Interval 1: TIME _____ HR _____ P _____
Interval 2: TIME _____ HR _____ P _____
Interval 3: TIME _____ HR _____ P _____
Interval 4: TIME _____ HR _____ P _____
Interval 5: TIME _____ HR _____ P _____

Workout Notes _____

Personal Notes _____

Thursday ▪ Date: ___/___/___

Waking Heart Rate _____

Standing Heart Rate _____

Waking Weight _____ Hours of Sleep _____

Quality of Sleep 1 2 3 4 5 6 7 8 9 10

Mood State 1 2 3 4 5 6 7 8 9 10

Goal _____

Workout _____

Specific Task _____

Actual Workout Time _____

Distance _____ Cadence _____ Power _____

Average Heart Rate _____

Interval 1: TIME _____ HR _____ P _____
Interval 2: TIME _____ HR _____ P _____
Interval 3: TIME _____ HR _____ P _____
Interval 4: TIME _____ HR _____ P _____
Interval 5: TIME _____ HR _____ P _____

Workout Notes _____

Personal Notes _____

Friday ▪ Date: ___/___/___

Waking Heart Rate _____

Standing Heart Rate _____

Waking Weight _____ Hours of Sleep _____

Quality of Sleep 1 2 3 4 5 6 7 8 9 10

Mood State 1 2 3 4 5 6 7 8 9 10

Goal _____

Workout _____

Specific Task _____

Actual Workout Time _____

Distance _____ Cadence _____ Power _____

Average Heart Rate _____

Interval 1: TIME _____ HR _____ P _____
Interval 2: TIME _____ HR _____ P _____
Interval 3: TIME _____ HR _____ P _____
Interval 4: TIME _____ HR _____ P _____
Interval 5: TIME _____ HR _____ P _____

Workout Notes _____

Personal Notes _____

Saturday ▪ Date: ___/___/___

Waking Heart Rate _____

Standing Heart Rate _____

Waking Weight _____ Hours of Sleep _____

Quality of Sleep 1 2 3 4 5 6 7 8 9 10

Mood State 1 2 3 4 5 6 7 8 9 10

Goal _____

Workout _____

Specific Task _____

Actual Workout Time _____

Distance _____ Cadence _____ Power _____

Average Heart Rate _____

Interval 1: TIME _____ HR _____ P _____
Interval 2: TIME _____ HR _____ P _____
Interval 3: TIME _____ HR _____ P _____
Interval 4: TIME _____ HR _____ P _____
Interval 5: TIME _____ HR _____ P _____

Workout Notes _____

Personal Notes _____

| Week # |

Sunday ■ Date: ___ / ___ / ___

Waking Heart Rate ___

Standing Heart Rate ___

Waking Weight ___ Hours of Sleep ___

Quality of Sleep 1 2 3 4 5 6 7 8 9 10

Mood State 1 2 3 4 5 6 7 8 9 10

Goal ___

Workout ___

Specific Task ___

Actual Workout Time ___

Distance ___ Cadence ___

Average Heart Rate ___ Power ___

Interval 1: TIME ___ HR ___ P ___

Interval 2: TIME ___ HR ___ P ___

Interval 3: TIME ___ HR ___ P ___

Interval 4: TIME ___ HR ___ P ___

Interval 5: TIME ___ HR ___ P ___

Workout Notes ___

Personal Notes ___

Weekly Summary

Hours of Cycling: ___ Year-to-Date: ___

Miles/Kilometers: ___ Year-to-Date: ___

Hours of Strength Training: ___ Year-to-Date: ___

Hours of Other Activities: ___ Year-to-Date: ___

___ Year-to-Date: ___

___ Year-to-Date: ___

___ Year-to-Date: ___

Total Training Hours: ___

Number of Workouts Planned: ___

Number of Workouts Completed: ___

Average Hours of Sleep: ___

Average Quality of Sleep: ___

Average Mood State: ___

Time Spent in Heart Rate/Power Ranges:

CTS RANGES	TIME	CTS RANGES	TIME	OTHER WORKOUTS	TIME
RecoveryMiles™		SteadyState™			
FoundationMiles™		ClimbingRepeats™			
EnduranceMiles™		Max Effort			
Tempo™					

Personal Notes: ___

Weekly Strength Training Record

Exercise	Date:									Date:								
	SET 1		SET 2		SET 3					SET 1		SET 2		SET 3				
	lbs.	reps	lbs.	reps	lbs.	reps				lbs.	reps	lbs.	reps	lbs.	reps			

Race Results

Race #1 _____ Date: ___ / ___ / ___

Time _____ Distance _____

Goal _____

Result _____

Average Heart Rate _____ Power _____

Food/Fluid Intake _____

Personal Notes _____

_____

_____

_____

Race #2 _____ Date: ___ / ___ / ___

Time _____ Distance _____

Goal _____

Result _____

Average Heart Rate _____ Power _____

Food/Fluid Intake _____

Personal Notes _____

_____

_____

_____

Monday ■ Date: ___ / ___ / ___

Waking Heart Rate _____

Standing Heart Rate _____

Waking Weight _____ Hours of Sleep _____

Quality of Sleep 1 2 3 4 5 6 7 8 9 10

Mood State 1 2 3 4 5 6 7 8 9 10

Goal _____

Workout _____

Specific Task _____

Actual Workout Time _____

Distance _____ Cadence _____

Average Heart Rate _____ Power _____

Interval 1: TIME _____ HR _____ P _____
Interval 2: TIME _____ HR _____ P _____
Interval 3: TIME _____ HR _____ P _____
Interval 4: TIME _____ HR _____ P _____
Interval 5: TIME _____ HR _____ P _____

Workout Notes _____

Personal Notes _____

Tuesday ■ Date: ___ / ___ / ___

Waking Heart Rate _____

Standing Heart Rate _____

Waking Weight _____ Hours of Sleep _____

Quality of Sleep 1 2 3 4 5 6 7 8 9 10

Mood State 1 2 3 4 5 6 7 8 9 10

Goal _____

Workout _____

Specific Task _____

Actual Workout Time _____

Distance _____ Cadence _____

Average Heart Rate _____ Power _____

Interval 1: TIME _____ HR _____ P _____
Interval 2: TIME _____ HR _____ P _____
Interval 3: TIME _____ HR _____ P _____
Interval 4: TIME _____ HR _____ P _____
Interval 5: TIME _____ HR _____ P _____

Workout Notes _____

Personal Notes _____

Wednesday ■ Date: ___ / ___ / ___

Waking Heart Rate _____

Standing Heart Rate _____

Waking Weight _____ Hours of Sleep _____

Quality of Sleep 1 2 3 4 5 6 7 8 9 10

Mood State 1 2 3 4 5 6 7 8 9 10

Goal _____

Workout _____

Specific Task _____

Actual Workout Time _____

Distance _____ Cadence _____

Average Heart Rate _____ Power _____

Interval 1: TIME _____ HR _____ P _____
Interval 2: TIME _____ HR _____ P _____
Interval 3: TIME _____ HR _____ P _____
Interval 4: TIME _____ HR _____ P _____
Interval 5: TIME _____ HR _____ P _____

Workout Notes _____

Personal Notes _____

Week #

Thursday ▪ Date: ___ / ___ / ___

Waking Heart Rate ___
Standing Heart Rate ___
Waking Weight ___ Hours of Sleep ___
Quality of Sleep 1 2 3 4 5 6 7 8 9 10

Mood State 1 2 3 4 5 6 7 8 9 10

Goal ___
Workout ___
Specific Task ___
Actual Workout Time ___
Distance ___ Cadence ___
Average Heart Rate ___ Power ___

Interval 1: TIME ___ HR ___ P ___
Interval 2: TIME ___ HR ___ P ___
Interval 3: TIME ___ HR ___ P ___
Interval 4: TIME ___ HR ___ P ___
Interval 5: TIME ___ HR ___ P ___

Workout Notes ___

Personal Notes ___

Friday ▪ Date: ___ / ___ / ___

Waking Heart Rate ___
Standing Heart Rate ___
Waking Weight ___ Hours of Sleep ___
Quality of Sleep 1 2 3 4 5 6 7 8 9 10

Mood State 1 2 3 4 5 6 7 8 9 10

Goal ___
Workout ___
Specific Task ___
Actual Workout Time ___
Distance ___ Cadence ___
Average Heart Rate ___ Power ___

Interval 1: TIME ___ HR ___ P ___
Interval 2: TIME ___ HR ___ P ___
Interval 3: TIME ___ HR ___ P ___
Interval 4: TIME ___ HR ___ P ___
Interval 5: TIME ___ HR ___ P ___

Workout Notes ___

Personal Notes ___

Saturday ▪ Date: ___ / ___ / ___

Waking Heart Rate ___
Standing Heart Rate ___
Waking Weight ___ Hours of Sleep ___
Quality of Sleep 1 2 3 4 5 6 7 8 9 10

Mood State 1 2 3 4 5 6 7 8 9 10

Goal ___
Workout ___
Specific Task ___
Actual Workout Time ___
Distance ___ Cadence ___
Average Heart Rate ___ Power ___

Interval 1: TIME ___ HR ___ P ___
Interval 2: TIME ___ HR ___ P ___
Interval 3: TIME ___ HR ___ P ___
Interval 4: TIME ___ HR ___ P ___
Interval 5: TIME ___ HR ___ P ___

Workout Notes ___

Personal Notes ___

Sunday ■ Date: ___ / ___ / ___

Waking Heart Rate _____

Standing Heart Rate _____

Waking Weight _____ Hours of Sleep _____

Quality of Sleep 1 2 3 4 5 6 7 8 9 10

Mood State 1 2 3 4 5 6 7 8 9 10

Goal _____

Workout _____

Specific Task _____

Actual Workout Time _____

Distance _____ Cadence _____

Average Heart Rate _____ Power _____

Interval 1: TIME _____ HR _____ P _____

Interval 2: TIME _____ HR _____ P _____

Interval 3: TIME _____ HR _____ P _____

Interval 4: TIME _____ HR _____ P _____

Interval 5: TIME _____ HR _____ P _____

Workout Notes _____

Personal Notes _____

Weekly Summary

Hours of Cycling: _____ Year-to-Date: _____

Miles/Kilometers: _____ Year-to-Date: _____

Hours of Strength Training: _____ Year-to-Date: _____

Hours of Other Activities: _____ Year-to-Date: _____

_____ Year-to-Date: _____

_____ Year-to-Date: _____

_____ Year-to-Date: _____

_____ Year-to-Date: _____

Total Training Hours: _____

Number of Workouts Planned: _____

Number of Workouts Completed: _____

Average Hours of Sleep: _____

Average Quality of Sleep: _____

Average Mood State: _____

Time Spent in Heart Rate/Power Ranges:

CTS RANGES	TIME	CTS RANGES	TIME	OTHER WORKOUTS	TIME
RecoveryMiles™		SteadyState™			
FoundationMiles™		ClimbingRepeats™			
EnduranceMiles™		Max Effort			
Tempo™					

Personal Notes: _____

Weekly Strength Training Record

Exercise	Date:						Date:						Date:					
	SET 1		SET 2		SET 3		SET 1		SET 2		SET 3		SET 1		SET 2		SET 3	
	lbs.	reps	lbs.	reps	lbs.	reps	lbs.	reps	lbs.	reps	lbs.	reps	lbs.	reps	lbs.	reps	lbs.	reps

Race Results

Race #1 _____ Date: ___/___/___

Time _____ Distance _____

Goal _____

Result _____

Average Heart Rate _____ Power _____

Food/Fluid Intake _____

Personal Notes _____

_____

_____

Race #2 _____ Date: ___/___/___

Time _____ Distance _____

Goal _____

Result _____

Average Heart Rate _____ Power _____

Food/Fluid Intake _____

Personal Notes _____

_____

_____

Week #		Goal:

Monday ■ Date: ___ / ___ / ___

Waking Heart Rate _____

Standing Heart Rate _____

Waking Weight _____ Hours of Sleep _____

Quality of Sleep 1 2 3 4 5 6 7 8 9 10

Mood State 1 2 3 4 5 6 7 8 9 10

Goal _____

Workout _____

Specific Task _____

Actual Workout Time _____

Distance _____ Cadence _____

Average Heart Rate _____ Power _____

Interval 1: TIME _____ HR _____ P _____

Interval 2: TIME _____ HR _____ P _____

Interval 3: TIME _____ HR _____ P _____

Interval 4: TIME _____ HR _____ P _____

Interval 5: TIME _____ HR _____ P _____

Workout Notes _____

Personal Notes _____

Tuesday ■ Date: ___ / ___ / ___

Waking Heart Rate _____

Standing Heart Rate _____

Waking Weight _____ Hours of Sleep _____

Quality of Sleep 1 2 3 4 5 6 7 8 9 10

Mood State 1 2 3 4 5 6 7 8 9 10

Goal _____

Workout _____

Specific Task _____

Actual Workout Time _____

Distance _____ Cadence _____

Average Heart Rate _____ Power _____

Interval 1: TIME _____ HR _____ P _____

Interval 2: TIME _____ HR _____ P _____

Interval 3: TIME _____ HR _____ P _____

Interval 4: TIME _____ HR _____ P _____

Interval 5: TIME _____ HR _____ P _____

Workout Notes _____

Personal Notes _____

Wednesday ■ Date: ___ / ___ / ___

Waking Heart Rate _____

Standing Heart Rate _____

Waking Weight _____ Hours of Sleep _____

Quality of Sleep 1 2 3 4 5 6 7 8 9 10

Mood State 1 2 3 4 5 6 7 8 9 10

Goal _____

Workout _____

Specific Task _____

Actual Workout Time _____

Distance _____ Cadence _____

Average Heart Rate _____ Power _____

Interval 1: TIME _____ HR _____ P _____

Interval 2: TIME _____ HR _____ P _____

Interval 3: TIME _____ HR _____ P _____

Interval 4: TIME _____ HR _____ P _____

Interval 5: TIME _____ HR _____ P _____

Workout Notes _____

Personal Notes _____

Thursday ■ Date: ___ / ___ / ___

Waking Heart Rate _____

Standing Heart Rate _____

Waking Weight _____ Hours of Sleep _____

Quality of Sleep   1 2 3 4 5 6 7 8 9 10

Mood State   1 2 3 4 5 6 7 8 9 10

Goal _____

Workout _____

Specific Task _____

Actual Workout Time _____

Distance _____ Cadence _____

Average Heart Rate _____ Power _____

Interval 1: TIME _____ HR _____ P _____

Interval 2: TIME _____ HR _____ P _____

Interval 3: TIME _____ HR _____ P _____

Interval 4: TIME _____ HR _____ P _____

Interval 5: TIME _____ HR _____ P _____

Workout Notes _____

Personal Notes _____

Friday ■ Date: ___ / ___ / ___

Waking Heart Rate _____

Standing Heart Rate _____

Waking Weight _____ Hours of Sleep _____

Quality of Sleep   1 2 3 4 5 6 7 8 9 10

Mood State   1 2 3 4 5 6 7 8 9 10

Goal _____

Workout _____

Specific Task _____

Actual Workout Time _____

Distance _____ Cadence _____

Average Heart Rate _____ Power _____

Interval 1: TIME _____ HR _____ P _____

Interval 2: TIME _____ HR _____ P _____

Interval 3: TIME _____ HR _____ P _____

Interval 4: TIME _____ HR _____ P _____

Interval 5: TIME _____ HR _____ P _____

Workout Notes _____

Personal Notes _____

Saturday ■ Date: ___ / ___ / ___

Waking Heart Rate _____

Standing Heart Rate _____

Waking Weight _____ Hours of Sleep _____

Quality of Sleep   1 2 3 4 5 6 7 8 9 10

Mood State   1 2 3 4 5 6 7 8 9 10

Goal _____

Workout _____

Specific Task _____

Actual Workout Time _____

Distance _____ Cadence _____

Average Heart Rate _____ Power _____

Interval 1: TIME _____ HR _____ P _____

Interval 2: TIME _____ HR _____ P _____

Interval 3: TIME _____ HR _____ P _____

Interval 4: TIME _____ HR _____ P _____

Interval 5: TIME _____ HR _____ P _____

Workout Notes _____

Personal Notes _____

Week # _____

Sunday ■ Date: ___ / ___ / ___

Waking Heart Rate _____

Standing Heart Rate _____

Waking Weight _____ Hours of Sleep _____

Quality of Sleep 1 2 3 4 5 6 7 8 9 10

Mood State 1 2 3 4 5 6 7 8 9 10

Goal _____

Workout _____

Specific Task _____

Actual Workout Time _____

Distance _____ Cadence _____

Average Heart Rate _____ Power _____

Interval 1: TIME _____ HR _____ P _____

Interval 2: TIME _____ HR _____ P _____

Interval 3: TIME _____ HR _____ P _____

Interval 4: TIME _____ HR _____ P _____

Interval 5: TIME _____ HR _____ P _____

Workout Notes _____

Personal Notes _____

Weekly Summary

Hours of Cycling: _____ Year-to-Date: _____

Miles/Kilometers: _____ Year-to-Date: _____

Hours of Strength Training: _____ Year-to-Date: _____

Hours of Other Activities: _____ Year-to-Date: _____

_____ Year-to-Date: _____

_____ Year-to-Date: _____

_____ Year-to-Date: _____

_____ Year-to-Date: _____

Total Training Hours: _____

Number of Workouts Planned: _____

Number of Workouts Completed: _____

Average Hours of Sleep: _____

Average Quality of Sleep: _____

Average Mood State: _____

Time Spent in Heart Rate/Power Ranges:

CTS RANGES	TIME	CTS RANGES	TIME	OTHER WORKOUTS	TIME
RecoveryMiles™		SteadyState™			
FoundationMiles™		ClimbingRepeats™			
EnduranceMiles™		Max Effort			
Tempo™					

Personal Notes: _____

Weekly Strength Training Record

Race Results

Exercise	Date:			Date:			Date:		
	SET 1 lbs./reps	SET 2 lbs./reps	SET 3 lbs./reps	SET 1 lbs./reps	SET 2 lbs./reps	SET 3 lbs./reps	SET 1 lbs./reps	SET 2 lbs./reps	SET 3 lbs./reps

Race #1 _____ Date: ___/___/___

Time _____ Distance _____

Goal _____

Result _____

Average Heart Rate _____ Power _____

Food/Fluid Intake _____

Personal Notes _____

Race #2 _____ Date: ___/___/___

Time _____ Distance _____

Goal _____

Result _____

Average Heart Rate _____ Power _____

Food/Fluid Intake _____

Personal Notes _____

Week # _____   Goal: _____

Monday ■ Date: ___ / ___ / ___

Waking Heart Rate _____

Standing Heart Rate _____

Waking Weight _____ Hours of Sleep _____

Quality of Sleep 1 2 3 4 5 6 7 8 9 10

Mood State 1 2 3 4 5 6 7 8 9 10

Goal _____

Workout _____

Specific Task _____

Actual Workout Time _____

Distance _____ Cadence _____

Average Heart Rate _____ Power _____

Interval 1: TIME _____ HR _____ P _____
Interval 2: TIME _____ HR _____ P _____
Interval 3: TIME _____ HR _____ P _____
Interval 4: TIME _____ HR _____ P _____
Interval 5: TIME _____ HR _____ P _____

Workout Notes _____

Personal Notes _____

Tuesday ■ Date: ___ / ___ / ___

Waking Heart Rate _____

Standing Heart Rate _____

Waking Weight _____ Hours of Sleep _____

Quality of Sleep 1 2 3 4 5 6 7 8 9 10

Mood State 1 2 3 4 5 6 7 8 9 10

Goal _____

Workout _____

Specific Task _____

Actual Workout Time _____

Distance _____ Cadence _____

Average Heart Rate _____ Power _____

Interval 1: TIME _____ HR _____ P _____
Interval 2: TIME _____ HR _____ P _____
Interval 3: TIME _____ HR _____ P _____
Interval 4: TIME _____ HR _____ P _____
Interval 5: TIME _____ HR _____ P _____

Workout Notes _____

Personal Notes _____

Wednesday ■ Date: ___ / ___ / ___

Waking Heart Rate _____

Standing Heart Rate _____

Waking Weight _____ Hours of Sleep _____

Quality of Sleep 1 2 3 4 5 6 7 8 9 10

Mood State 1 2 3 4 5 6 7 8 9 10

Goal _____

Workout _____

Specific Task _____

Actual Workout Time _____

Distance _____ Cadence _____

Average Heart Rate _____ Power _____

Interval 1: TIME _____ HR _____ P _____
Interval 2: TIME _____ HR _____ P _____
Interval 3: TIME _____ HR _____ P _____
Interval 4: TIME _____ HR _____ P _____
Interval 5: TIME _____ HR _____ P _____

Workout Notes _____

Personal Notes _____

Thursday ■ Date: ___ / ___ / ___

Waking Heart Rate _____

Standing Heart Rate _____

Waking Weight _____ Hours of Sleep _____

Quality of Sleep 1 2 3 4 5 6 7 8 9 10

Mood State 1 2 3 4 5 6 7 8 9 10

Goal _____

Workout _____

Specific Task _____

Actual Workout Time _____

Distance _____ Cadence _____

Average Heart Rate _____ Power _____

Interval 1: TIME _____ HR _____ P _____
Interval 2: TIME _____ HR _____ P _____
Interval 3: TIME _____ HR _____ P _____
Interval 4: TIME _____ HR _____ P _____
Interval 5: TIME _____ HR _____ P _____

Workout Notes _____

Personal Notes _____

Friday ■ Date: ___ / ___ / ___

Waking Heart Rate _____

Standing Heart Rate _____

Waking Weight _____ Hours of Sleep _____

Quality of Sleep 1 2 3 4 5 6 7 8 9 10

Mood State 1 2 3 4 5 6 7 8 9 10

Goal _____

Workout _____

Specific Task _____

Actual Workout Time _____

Distance _____ Cadence _____

Average Heart Rate _____ Power _____

Interval 1: TIME _____ HR _____ P _____
Interval 2: TIME _____ HR _____ P _____
Interval 3: TIME _____ HR _____ P _____
Interval 4: TIME _____ HR _____ P _____
Interval 5: TIME _____ HR _____ P _____

Workout Notes _____

Personal Notes _____

Saturday ■ Date: ___ / ___ / ___

Waking Heart Rate _____

Standing Heart Rate _____

Waking Weight _____ Hours of Sleep _____

Quality of Sleep 1 2 3 4 5 6 7 8 9 10

Mood State 1 2 3 4 5 6 7 8 9 10

Goal _____

Workout _____

Specific Task _____

Actual Workout Time _____

Distance _____ Cadence _____

Average Heart Rate _____ Power _____

Interval 1: TIME _____ HR _____ P _____
Interval 2: TIME _____ HR _____ P _____
Interval 3: TIME _____ HR _____ P _____
Interval 4: TIME _____ HR _____ P _____
Interval 5: TIME _____ HR _____ P _____

Workout Notes _____

Personal Notes _____

| Week # |

Sunday ■ Date: ___ / ___ / ___

Waking Heart Rate _____

Standing Heart Rate _____

Waking Weight _____ Hours of Sleep _____

Quality of Sleep 1 2 3 4 5 6 7 8 9 10

Mood State 1 2 3 4 5 6 7 8 9 10

Goal _____

Workout _____

Specific Task _____

Actual Workout Time _____

Distance _____ Cadence _____

Average Heart Rate _____ Power _____

Interval 1:	TIME ___	HR ___	P ___
Interval 2:	TIME ___	HR ___	P ___
Interval 3:	TIME ___	HR ___	P ___
Interval 4:	TIME ___	HR ___	P ___
Interval 5:	TIME ___	HR ___	P ___

Workout Notes _____

Personal Notes _____

Weekly Summary

Hours of Cycling: _____ Year-to-Date: _____

Miles/Kilometers: _____ Year-to-Date: _____

Hours of Strength Training: _____ Year-to-Date: _____

Hours of Other Activities: _____ Year-to-Date: _____

_____ Year-to-Date: _____

_____ Year-to-Date: _____

_____ Year-to-Date: _____

_____ Year-to-Date: _____

Total Training Hours: _____

Number of Workouts Planned: _____

Number of Workouts Completed: _____

Average Hours of Sleep: _____

Average Quality of Sleep: _____

Average Mood State: _____

Time Spent in Heart Rate/Power Ranges:

CTS RANGES	TIME	CTS RANGES	TIME	OTHER WORKOUTS	TIME
RecoveryMiles™		SteadyState™			
FoundationMiles™		ClimbingRepeats™			
EnduranceMiles™		Max Effort			
Tempo™					

Personal Notes: _____

Week # _____   **Weekly Strength Training Record**

Exercise	Date:	SET 1 lbs. / reps	SET 2 lbs. / reps	SET 3 lbs. / reps	Date:	SET 1 lbs. / reps	SET 2 lbs. / reps	SET 3 lbs. / reps	Date:	SET 1 lbs. / reps	SET 2 lbs. / reps	SET 3 lbs. / reps

Race Results

Race #1 _____   Date: ___ / ___ / ___

Time _____   Distance _____

Goal _____

Result _____

Average Heart Rate _____   Power _____

Food/Fluid Intake _____

Personal Notes _____

_____

Race #2 _____   Date: ___ / ___ / ___

Time _____   Distance _____

Goal _____

Result _____

Average Heart Rate _____   Power _____

Food/Fluid Intake _____

Personal Notes _____

_____

Week #	Goal: _____

Monday ■ Date: ___/___/___

Waking Heart Rate _____
Standing Heart Rate _____
Waking Weight _____ Hours of Sleep _____
Quality of Sleep 1 2 3 4 5 6 7 8 9 10

Mood State 1 2 3 4 5 6 7 8 9 10

Goal _____
Workout _____
Specific Task _____
Actual Workout Time _____
Distance _____ Cadence _____
Average Heart Rate _____ Power _____

Interval 1:	TIME ____	HR ____	P ____
Interval 2:	TIME ____	HR ____	P ____
Interval 3:	TIME ____	HR ____	P ____
Interval 4:	TIME ____	HR ____	P ____
Interval 5:	TIME ____	HR ____	P ____

Workout Notes _____

Personal Notes _____

Tuesday ■ Date: ___/___/___

Waking Heart Rate _____
Standing Heart Rate _____
Waking Weight _____ Hours of Sleep _____
Quality of Sleep 1 2 3 4 5 6 7 8 9 10

Mood State 1 2 3 4 5 6 7 8 9 10

Goal _____
Workout _____
Specific Task _____
Actual Workout Time _____
Distance _____ Cadence _____
Average Heart Rate _____ Power _____

Interval 1:	TIME ____	HR ____	P ____
Interval 2:	TIME ____	HR ____	P ____
Interval 3:	TIME ____	HR ____	P ____
Interval 4:	TIME ____	HR ____	P ____
Interval 5:	TIME ____	HR ____	P ____

Workout Notes _____

Personal Notes _____

Wednesday ■ Date: ___/___/___

Waking Heart Rate _____
Standing Heart Rate _____
Waking Weight _____ Hours of Sleep _____
Quality of Sleep 1 2 3 4 5 6 7 8 9 10

Mood State 1 2 3 4 5 6 7 8 9 10

Goal _____
Workout _____
Specific Task _____
Actual Workout Time _____
Distance _____ Cadence _____
Average Heart Rate _____ Power _____

Interval 1:	TIME ____	HR ____	P ____
Interval 2:	TIME ____	HR ____	P ____
Interval 3:	TIME ____	HR ____	P ____
Interval 4:	TIME ____	HR ____	P ____
Interval 5:	TIME ____	HR ____	P ____

Workout Notes _____

Personal Notes _____

Thursday ■ Date: ___ / ___ / ___

Waking Heart Rate _____

Standing Heart Rate _____

Waking Weight _____ Hours of Sleep _____

Quality of Sleep 1 2 3 4 5 6 7 8 9 10

Mood State 1 2 3 4 5 6 7 8 9 10

Goal _____

Workout _____

Specific Task _____

Actual Workout Time _____

Distance _____ Cadence _____

Average Heart Rate _____ Power _____

Interval 1: TIME _____ HR _____ P _____
Interval 2: TIME _____ HR _____ P _____
Interval 3: TIME _____ HR _____ P _____
Interval 4: TIME _____ HR _____ P _____
Interval 5: TIME _____ HR _____ P _____

Workout Notes _____

Personal Notes _____

Friday ■ Date: ___ / ___ / ___

Waking Heart Rate _____

Standing Heart Rate _____

Waking Weight _____ Hours of Sleep _____

Quality of Sleep 1 2 3 4 5 6 7 8 9 10

Mood State 1 2 3 4 5 6 7 8 9 10

Goal _____

Workout _____

Specific Task _____

Actual Workout Time _____

Distance _____ Cadence _____

Average Heart Rate _____ Power _____

Interval 1: TIME _____ HR _____ P _____
Interval 2: TIME _____ HR _____ P _____
Interval 3: TIME _____ HR _____ P _____
Interval 4: TIME _____ HR _____ P _____
Interval 5: TIME _____ HR _____ P _____

Workout Notes _____

Personal Notes _____

Saturday ■ Date: ___ / ___ / ___

Waking Heart Rate _____

Standing Heart Rate _____

Waking Weight _____ Hours of Sleep _____

Quality of Sleep 1 2 3 4 5 6 7 8 9 10

Mood State 1 2 3 4 5 6 7 8 9 10

Goal _____

Workout _____

Specific Task _____

Actual Workout Time _____

Distance _____ Cadence _____

Average Heart Rate _____ Power _____

Interval 1: TIME _____ HR _____ P _____
Interval 2: TIME _____ HR _____ P _____
Interval 3: TIME _____ HR _____ P _____
Interval 4: TIME _____ HR _____ P _____
Interval 5: TIME _____ HR _____ P _____

Workout Notes _____

Personal Notes _____

Sunday ■ Date: ___ / ___ / ___

Waking Heart Rate _____

Standing Heart Rate _____

Waking Weight _____ Hours of Sleep _____

Quality of Sleep 1 2 3 4 5 6 7 8 9 10

Mood State 1 2 3 4 5 6 7 8 9 10

Goal _____

Workout _____

Specific Task _____

Actual Workout Time _____

Distance _____ Cadence _____

Average Heart Rate _____ Power _____

Interval 1:	TIME ___	HR ___	P ___
Interval 2:	TIME ___	HR ___	P ___
Interval 3:	TIME ___	HR ___	P ___
Interval 4:	TIME ___	HR ___	P ___
Interval 5:	TIME ___	HR ___	P ___

Workout Notes _____

Personal Notes _____

Weekly Summary

Hours of Cycling: _____ Year-to-Date: _____

Miles/Kilometers: _____ Year-to-Date: _____

Hours of Strength Training: _____ Year-to-Date: _____

Hours of Other Activities: _____ Year-to-Date: _____

_____ Year-to-Date: _____

_____ Year-to-Date: _____

Total Training Hours: _____

Number of Workouts Planned: _____

Number of Workouts Completed: _____

Average Hours of Sleep: _____

Average Quality of Sleep: _____

Average Mood State: _____

Time Spent in Heart Rate/Power Ranges:

CTS RANGES	TIME	CTS RANGES	TIME	OTHER WORKOUTS	TIME
RecoveryMiles™	___	SteadyState™	___		___
FoundationMiles™	___	ClimbingRepeats™	___		___
EnduranceMiles™	___	Max Effort	___		
Tempo™	___				

Personal Notes: _____

Week # _____

Weekly Strength Training Record

Exercise	Date:						Date:					
	SET 1 lbs. / reps		SET 2 lbs. / reps		SET 3 lbs. / reps		SET 1 lbs. / reps		SET 2 lbs. / reps		SET 3 lbs. / reps	

Race Results

Race #1 _____ Date: ___/___/___

Time _____ Distance _____

Goal _____

Result _____

Average Heart Rate _____ Power _____

Food/Fluid Intake _____

Personal Notes _____
_____
_____

Race #2 _____ Date: ___/___/___

Time _____ Distance _____

Goal _____

Result _____

Average Heart Rate _____ Power _____

Food/Fluid Intake _____

Personal Notes _____
_____
_____

| Week # _____ | Goal: _____ |

Monday ▪ Date: ___ / ___ / ___

Waking Heart Rate _____

Standing Heart Rate _____

Waking Weight _____ Hours of Sleep _____

Quality of Sleep 1 2 3 4 5 6 7 8 9 10

Mood State 1 2 3 4 5 6 7 8 9 10

Goal _____

Workout _____

Specific Task _____

Actual Workout Time _____

Distance _____ Cadence _____

Average Heart Rate _____ Power _____

Interval 1: TIME _____ HR _____ P _____

Interval 2: TIME _____ HR _____ P _____

Interval 3: TIME _____ HR _____ P _____

Interval 4: TIME _____ HR _____ P _____

Interval 5: TIME _____ HR _____ P _____

Workout Notes _____

Personal Notes _____

Tuesday ▪ Date: ___ / ___ / ___

Waking Heart Rate _____

Standing Heart Rate _____

Waking Weight _____ Hours of Sleep _____

Quality of Sleep 1 2 3 4 5 6 7 8 9 10

Mood State 1 2 3 4 5 6 7 8 9 10

Goal _____

Workout _____

Specific Task _____

Actual Workout Time _____

Distance _____ Cadence _____

Average Heart Rate _____ Power _____

Interval 1: TIME _____ HR _____ P _____

Interval 2: TIME _____ HR _____ P _____

Interval 3: TIME _____ HR _____ P _____

Interval 4: TIME _____ HR _____ P _____

Interval 5: TIME _____ HR _____ P _____

Workout Notes _____

Personal Notes _____

Wednesday ▪ Date: ___ / ___ / ___

Waking Heart Rate _____

Standing Heart Rate _____

Waking Weight _____ Hours of Sleep _____

Quality of Sleep 1 2 3 4 5 6 7 8 9 10

Mood State 1 2 3 4 5 6 7 8 9 10

Goal _____

Workout _____

Specific Task _____

Actual Workout Time _____

Distance _____ Cadence _____

Average Heart Rate _____ Power _____

Interval 1: TIME _____ HR _____ P _____

Interval 2: TIME _____ HR _____ P _____

Interval 3: TIME _____ HR _____ P _____

Interval 4: TIME _____ HR _____ P _____

Interval 5: TIME _____ HR _____ P _____

Workout Notes _____

Personal Notes _____

Thursday ■ Date: ___ / ___ / ___

Waking Heart Rate _____

Standing Heart Rate _____

Waking Weight _____ Hours of Sleep _____

Quality of Sleep 1 2 3 4 5 6 7 8 9 10

Mood State 1 2 3 4 5 6 7 8 9 10

Goal _____

Workout _____

Specific Task _____

Actual Workout Time _____

Distance _____ Cadence _____

Average Heart Rate _____ Power _____

Interval 1: TIME _____ HR _____ P _____

Interval 2: TIME _____ HR _____ P _____

Interval 3: TIME _____ HR _____ P _____

Interval 4: TIME _____ HR _____ P _____

Interval 5: TIME _____ HR _____ P _____

Workout Notes _____

Personal Notes _____

Friday ■ Date: ___ / ___ / ___

Waking Heart Rate _____

Standing Heart Rate _____

Waking Weight _____ Hours of Sleep _____

Quality of Sleep 1 2 3 4 5 6 7 8 9 10

Mood State 1 2 3 4 5 6 7 8 9 10

Goal _____

Workout _____

Specific Task _____

Actual Workout Time _____

Distance _____ Cadence _____

Average Heart Rate _____ Power _____

Interval 1: TIME _____ HR _____ P _____

Interval 2: TIME _____ HR _____ P _____

Interval 3: TIME _____ HR _____ P _____

Interval 4: TIME _____ HR _____ P _____

Interval 5: TIME _____ HR _____ P _____

Workout Notes _____

Personal Notes _____

Saturday ■ Date: ___ / ___ / ___

Waking Heart Rate _____

Standing Heart Rate _____

Waking Weight _____ Hours of Sleep _____

Quality of Sleep 1 2 3 4 5 6 7 8 9 10

Mood State 1 2 3 4 5 6 7 8 9 10

Goal _____

Workout _____

Specific Task _____

Actual Workout Time _____

Distance _____ Cadence _____

Average Heart Rate _____ Power _____

Interval 1: TIME _____ HR _____ P _____

Interval 2: TIME _____ HR _____ P _____

Interval 3: TIME _____ HR _____ P _____

Interval 4: TIME _____ HR _____ P _____

Interval 5: TIME _____ HR _____ P _____

Workout Notes _____

Personal Notes _____

Sunday ■ Date: ___ / ___ / ___

Waking Heart Rate _____

Standing Heart Rate _____

Waking Weight _____ Hours of Sleep _____

Quality of Sleep 1 2 3 4 5 6 7 8 9 10

Mood State 1 2 3 4 5 6 7 8 9 10

Goal _____

Workout _____

Specific Task _____

Actual Workout Time _____

Distance _____ Cadence _____

Average Heart Rate _____ Power _____

Interval 1:	TIME _____	HR _____ P _____
Interval 2:	TIME _____	HR _____ P _____
Interval 3:	TIME _____	HR _____ P _____
Interval 4:	TIME _____	HR _____ P _____
Interval 5:	TIME _____	HR _____ P _____

Workout Notes _____

Personal Notes _____

Weekly Summary

Hours of Cycling: _____ Year-to-Date: _____

Miles/Kilometers: _____ Year-to-Date: _____

Hours of Strength Training: _____ Year-to-Date: _____

Hours of Other Activities: _____

_____ Year-to-Date: _____

_____ Year-to-Date: _____

_____ Year-to-Date: _____

Total Training Hours: _____

Number of Workouts Planned: _____

Number of Workouts Completed: _____

Average Hours of Sleep: _____

Average Quality of Sleep: _____

Average Mood State: _____

Time Spent in Heart Rate/Power Ranges:

CTS RANGES	TIME	CTS RANGES	TIME	OTHER WORKOUTS	TIME
RecoveryMiles™	_____	SteadyState™	_____	_____	_____
FoundationMiles™	_____	ClimbingRepeats™	_____	_____	_____
EnduranceMiles™	_____	Max Effort	_____	_____	_____
Tempo™	_____				

Personal Notes: _____

Weekly Strength Training Record

Race Results

Exercise	Date:						Date:						Date:					
	SET 1		SET 2		SET 3		SET 1		SET 2		SET 3		SET 1		SET 2		SET 3	
	lbs.	reps	lbs.	reps	lbs.	reps	lbs.	reps	lbs.	reps	lbs.	reps	lbs.	reps	lbs.	reps	lbs.	reps

Race #1 _____ Date: ___ / ___ / ___

Time _____ Distance _____

Goal _____

Result _____

Average Heart Rate _____ Power _____

Food/Fluid Intake _____

Personal Notes _____

Race #2 _____ Date: ___ / ___ / ___

Time _____ Distance _____

Goal _____

Result _____

Average Heart Rate _____ Power _____

Food/Fluid Intake _____

Personal Notes _____

Week # _____   Goal: _____

Monday ■ Date: ___/___/___

Waking Heart Rate _____
Standing Heart Rate _____
Waking Weight _____ Hours of Sleep _____
Quality of Sleep 1 2 3 4 5 6 7 8 9 10

Mood State 1 2 3 4 5 6 7 8 9 10

Goal _____
Workout _____
Specific Task _____
Actual Workout Time _____
Distance _____ Cadence _____
Average Heart Rate _____ Power _____

Interval 1: TIME _____ HR _____ P _____
Interval 2: TIME _____ HR _____ P _____
Interval 3: TIME _____ HR _____ P _____
Interval 4: TIME _____ HR _____ P _____
Interval 5: TIME _____ HR _____ P _____

Workout Notes _____

Personal Notes _____

Tuesday ■ Date: ___/___/___

Waking Heart Rate _____
Standing Heart Rate _____
Waking Weight _____ Hours of Sleep _____
Quality of Sleep 1 2 3 4 5 6 7 8 9 10

Mood State 1 2 3 4 5 6 7 8 9 10

Goal _____
Workout _____
Specific Task _____
Actual Workout Time _____
Distance _____ Cadence _____
Average Heart Rate _____ Power _____

Interval 1: TIME _____ HR _____ P _____
Interval 2: TIME _____ HR _____ P _____
Interval 3: TIME _____ HR _____ P _____
Interval 4: TIME _____ HR _____ P _____
Interval 5: TIME _____ HR _____ P _____

Workout Notes _____

Personal Notes _____

Wednesday ■ Date: ___/___/___

Waking Heart Rate _____
Standing Heart Rate _____
Waking Weight _____ Hours of Sleep _____
Quality of Sleep 1 2 3 4 5 6 7 8 9 10

Mood State 1 2 3 4 5 6 7 8 9 10

Goal _____
Workout _____
Specific Task _____
Actual Workout Time _____
Distance _____ Cadence _____
Average Heart Rate _____ Power _____

Interval 1: TIME _____ HR _____ P _____
Interval 2: TIME _____ HR _____ P _____
Interval 3: TIME _____ HR _____ P _____
Interval 4: TIME _____ HR _____ P _____
Interval 5: TIME _____ HR _____ P _____

Workout Notes _____

Personal Notes _____

Thursday ■ Date: ___ / ___ / ___

Waking Heart Rate _____

Standing Heart Rate _____

Waking Weight _____ Hours of Sleep _____

Quality of Sleep 1 2 3 4 5 6 7 8 9 10

Mood State 1 2 3 4 5 6 7 8 9 10

Goal _____

Workout _____

Specific Task _____

Actual Workout Time _____

Distance _____ Cadence _____

Average Heart Rate _____ Power _____

		HR	P
Interval 1:	TIME	HR ___	P ___
Interval 2:	TIME	HR ___	P ___
Interval 3:	TIME	HR ___	P ___
Interval 4:	TIME	HR ___	P ___
Interval 5:	TIME	HR ___	P ___

Workout Notes _____

Personal Notes _____

Friday ■ Date: ___ / ___ / ___

Waking Heart Rate _____

Standing Heart Rate _____

Waking Weight _____ Hours of Sleep _____

Quality of Sleep 1 2 3 4 5 6 7 8 9 10

Mood State 1 2 3 4 5 6 7 8 9 10

Goal _____

Workout _____

Specific Task _____

Actual Workout Time _____

Distance _____ Cadence _____

Average Heart Rate _____ Power _____

		HR	P
Interval 1:	TIME	HR ___	P ___
Interval 2:	TIME	HR ___	P ___
Interval 3:	TIME	HR ___	P ___
Interval 4:	TIME	HR ___	P ___
Interval 5:	TIME	HR ___	P ___

Workout Notes _____

Personal Notes _____

Saturday ■ Date: ___ / ___ / ___

Waking Heart Rate _____

Standing Heart Rate _____

Waking Weight _____ Hours of Sleep _____

Quality of Sleep 1 2 3 4 5 6 7 8 9 10

Mood State 1 2 3 4 5 6 7 8 9 10

Goal _____

Workout _____

Specific Task _____

Actual Workout Time _____

Distance _____ Cadence _____

Average Heart Rate _____ Power _____

		HR	P
Interval 1:	TIME	HR ___	P ___
Interval 2:	TIME	HR ___	P ___
Interval 3:	TIME	HR ___	P ___
Interval 4:	TIME	HR ___	P ___
Interval 5:	TIME	HR ___	P ___

Workout Notes _____

Personal Notes _____

| Week # | |

Sunday ■ Date: ___ / ___ / ___

Waking Heart Rate _____

Standing Heart Rate _____

Waking Weight _____ Hours of Sleep _____

Quality of Sleep 1 2 3 4 5 6 7 8 9 10

Mood State 1 2 3 4 5 6 7 8 9 10

Goal _____

Workout _____

Specific Task _____

Actual Workout Time _____

Distance _____ Cadence _____

Average Heart Rate _____ Power _____

Interval 1:	TIME	HR _____	P _____
Interval 2:	TIME	HR _____	P _____
Interval 3:	TIME	HR _____	P _____
Interval 4:	TIME	HR _____	P _____
Interval 5:	TIME	HR _____	P _____

Workout Notes _____

Personal Notes _____

Weekly Summary

Hours of Cycling: _____ Year-to-Date: _____

Miles/Kilometers: _____ Year-to-Date: _____

Hours of Strength Training: _____ Year-to-Date: _____

Hours of Other Activities: _____ Year-to-Date: _____

_____ Year-to-Date: _____

_____ Year-to-Date: _____

_____ Year-to-Date: _____

Total Training Hours: _____

Number of Workouts Planned: _____

Number of Workouts Completed: _____

Average Hours of Sleep: _____

Average Quality of Sleep: _____

Average Mood State: _____

Time Spent in Heart Rate/Power Ranges:

CTS RANGES	TIME	CTS RANGES	TIME	OTHER WORKOUTS	TIME
RecoveryMiles™		SteadyState™			
FoundationMiles™		ClimbingRepeats™			
EnduranceMiles™		Max Effort			
Tempo™					

Personal Notes: _____

Week # ____   Weekly Strength Training Record

Exercise	Date: ____						Date: ____						Date: ____					
	SET 1		SET 2		SET 3		SET 1		SET 2		SET 3		SET 1		SET 2		SET 3	
	lbs.	reps	lbs.	reps	lbs.	reps	lbs.	reps	lbs.	reps	lbs.	reps	lbs.	reps	lbs.	reps	lbs.	reps

Race Results

Race #1 _____   Date: ___/___/___

Time_____   Distance_____

Goal_____

Result_____

Average Heart Rate_____   Power_____

Food/Fluid Intake_____

Personal Notes_____

_____

_____

Race #2 _____   Date: ___/___/___

Time_____   Distance_____

Goal_____

Result_____

Average Heart Rate_____   Power_____

Food/Fluid Intake_____

Personal Notes_____

_____

_____

| 167 |

Week # _____   Goal: _____

Monday ■ Date: ___ / ___ / ___

Waking Heart Rate _____

Standing Heart Rate _____

Waking Weight _____ Hours of Sleep _____

Quality of Sleep 1 2 3 4 5 6 7 8 9 10

Mood State 1 2 3 4 5 6 7 8 9 10

Goal _____

Workout _____

Specific Task _____

Actual Workout Time _____

Distance _____ Cadence _____

Average Heart Rate _____ Power _____

Interval 1: TIME _____ HR _____ P _____

Interval 2: TIME _____ HR _____ P _____

Interval 3: TIME _____ HR _____ P _____

Interval 4: TIME _____ HR _____ P _____

Interval 5: TIME _____ HR _____ P _____

Workout Notes _____

Personal Notes _____

Tuesday ■ Date: ___ / ___ / ___

Waking Heart Rate _____

Standing Heart Rate _____

Waking Weight _____ Hours of Sleep _____

Quality of Sleep 1 2 3 4 5 6 7 8 9 10

Mood State 1 2 3 4 5 6 7 8 9 10

Goal _____

Workout _____

Specific Task _____

Actual Workout Time _____

Distance _____ Cadence _____

Average Heart Rate _____ Power _____

Interval 1: TIME _____ HR _____ P _____

Interval 2: TIME _____ HR _____ P _____

Interval 3: TIME _____ HR _____ P _____

Interval 4: TIME _____ HR _____ P _____

Interval 5: TIME _____ HR _____ P _____

Workout Notes _____

Personal Notes _____

Wednesday ■ Date: ___ / ___ / ___

Waking Heart Rate _____

Standing Heart Rate _____

Waking Weight _____ Hours of Sleep _____

Quality of Sleep 1 2 3 4 5 6 7 8 9 10

Mood State 1 2 3 4 5 6 7 8 9 10

Goal _____

Workout _____

Specific Task _____

Actual Workout Time _____

Distance _____ Cadence _____

Average Heart Rate _____ Power _____

Interval 1: TIME _____ HR _____ P _____

Interval 2: TIME _____ HR _____ P _____

Interval 3: TIME _____ HR _____ P _____

Interval 4: TIME _____ HR _____ P _____

Interval 5: TIME _____ HR _____ P _____

Workout Notes _____

Personal Notes _____

Thursday ■ Date: ___ / ___ / ___

Waking Heart Rate _____

Standing Heart Rate _____

Waking Weight _____ Hours of Sleep _____

Quality of Sleep   1 2 3 4 5 6 7 8 9 10

Mood State   1 2 3 4 5 6 7 8 9 10

Goal _____

Workout _____

Specific Task _____

Actual Workout Time _____

Distance _____ Cadence _____

Average Heart Rate _____ Power _____

Interval 1: TIME _____ HR _____ P _____

Interval 2: TIME _____ HR _____ P _____

Interval 3: TIME _____ HR _____ P _____

Interval 4: TIME _____ HR _____ P _____

Interval 5: TIME _____ HR _____ P _____

Workout Notes _____

Personal Notes _____

Friday ■ Date: ___ / ___ / ___

Waking Heart Rate _____

Standing Heart Rate _____

Waking Weight _____ Hours of Sleep _____

Quality of Sleep   1 2 3 4 5 6 7 8 9 10

Mood State   1 2 3 4 5 6 7 8 9 10

Goal _____

Workout _____

Specific Task _____

Actual Workout Time _____

Distance _____ Cadence _____

Average Heart Rate _____ Power _____

Interval 1: TIME _____ HR _____ P _____

Interval 2: TIME _____ HR _____ P _____

Interval 3: TIME _____ HR _____ P _____

Interval 4: TIME _____ HR _____ P _____

Interval 5: TIME _____ HR _____ P _____

Workout Notes _____

Personal Notes _____

Saturday ■ Date: ___ / ___ / ___

Waking Heart Rate _____

Standing Heart Rate _____

Waking Weight _____ Hours of Sleep _____

Quality of Sleep   1 2 3 4 5 6 7 8 9 10

Mood State   1 2 3 4 5 6 7 8 9 10

Goal _____

Workout _____

Specific Task _____

Actual Workout Time _____

Distance _____ Cadence _____

Average Heart Rate _____ Power _____

Interval 1: TIME _____ HR _____ P _____

Interval 2: TIME _____ HR _____ P _____

Interval 3: TIME _____ HR _____ P _____

Interval 4: TIME _____ HR _____ P _____

Interval 5: TIME _____ HR _____ P _____

Workout Notes _____

Personal Notes _____

Sunday ■ Date: ___ / ___ / ___

Waking Heart Rate _____

Standing Heart Rate _____

Waking Weight _____ Hours of Sleep _____

Quality of Sleep 1 2 3 4 5 6 7 8 9 10

Mood State 1 2 3 4 5 6 7 8 9 10

Goal _____

Workout _____

Specific Task _____

Actual Workout Time _____

Distance _____ Cadence _____

Average Heart Rate _____ Power _____

Interval 1: TIME _____ HR _____ P _____

Interval 2: TIME _____ HR _____ P _____

Interval 3: TIME _____ HR _____ P _____

Interval 4: TIME _____ HR _____ P _____

Interval 5: TIME _____ HR _____ P _____

Workout Notes _____

Personal Notes _____

Weekly Summary

Hours of Cycling: _____ Year-to-Date: _____

Miles/Kilometers: _____ Year-to-Date: _____

Hours of Strength Training: _____ Year-to-Date: _____

Hours of Other Activities: _____

_____ Year-to-Date: _____

_____ Year-to-Date: _____

_____ Year-to-Date: _____

_____ Year-to-Date: _____

Total Training Hours: _____

Number of Workouts Planned: _____

Number of Workouts Completed: _____

Average Hours of Sleep: _____

Average Quality of Sleep: _____

Average Mood State: _____

Time Spent in Heart Rate/Power Ranges:

CTS RANGES	TIME	CTS RANGES	TIME	OTHER WORKOUTS	TIME
RecoveryMiles™		SteadyState™			
FoundationMiles™		ClimbingRepeats™			
EnduranceMiles™		Max Effort			
Tempo™					

Personal Notes: _____

Weekly Strength Training Record

Exercise	Date:						Date:						Date:					
	SET 1		SET 2		SET 3		SET 1		SET 2		SET 3		SET 1		SET 2		SET 3	
	lbs.	reps	lbs.	reps	lbs.	reps	lbs.	reps	lbs.	reps	lbs.	reps	lbs.	reps	lbs.	reps	lbs.	reps

Race Results

Race #1 _____ Date: ___/___/___

Time _____ Distance _____

Goal _____

Result _____

Average Heart Rate _____ Power _____

Food/Fluid Intake _____

Personal Notes _____

_____

_____

_____

Race #2 _____ Date: ___/___/___

Time _____ Distance _____

Goal _____

Result _____

Average Heart Rate _____ Power _____

Food/Fluid Intake _____

Personal Notes _____

_____

_____

_____

Week # _____   Goal: _____

Monday ■ Date: ___ / ___ / ___

Waking Heart Rate _____

Standing Heart Rate _____

Waking Weight _____ Hours of Sleep _____

Quality of Sleep 1 2 3 4 5 6 7 8 9 10

Mood State 1 2 3 4 5 6 7 8 9 10

Goal _____

Workout _____

Specific Task _____

Actual Workout Time _____

Distance _____ Cadence _____

Average Heart Rate _____ Power _____

Interval 1: TIME _____ HR _____ P _____
Interval 2: TIME _____ HR _____ P _____
Interval 3: TIME _____ HR _____ P _____
Interval 4: TIME _____ HR _____ P _____
Interval 5: TIME _____ HR _____ P _____

Workout Notes _____

Personal Notes _____

Tuesday ■ Date: ___ / ___ / ___

Waking Heart Rate _____

Standing Heart Rate _____

Waking Weight _____ Hours of Sleep _____

Quality of Sleep 1 2 3 4 5 6 7 8 9 10

Mood State 1 2 3 4 5 6 7 8 9 10

Goal _____

Workout _____

Specific Task _____

Actual Workout Time _____

Distance _____ Cadence _____

Average Heart Rate _____ Power _____

Interval 1: TIME _____ HR _____ P _____
Interval 2: TIME _____ HR _____ P _____
Interval 3: TIME _____ HR _____ P _____
Interval 4: TIME _____ HR _____ P _____
Interval 5: TIME _____ HR _____ P _____

Workout Notes _____

Personal Notes _____

Wednesday ■ Date: ___ / ___ / ___

Waking Heart Rate _____

Standing Heart Rate _____

Waking Weight _____ Hours of Sleep _____

Quality of Sleep 1 2 3 4 5 6 7 8 9 10

Mood State 1 2 3 4 5 6 7 8 9 10

Goal _____

Workout _____

Specific Task _____

Actual Workout Time _____

Distance _____ Cadence _____

Average Heart Rate _____ Power _____

Interval 1: TIME _____ HR _____ P _____
Interval 2: TIME _____ HR _____ P _____
Interval 3: TIME _____ HR _____ P _____
Interval 4: TIME _____ HR _____ P _____
Interval 5: TIME _____ HR _____ P _____

Workout Notes _____

Personal Notes _____

Thursday ■ Date: ___ / ___ / ___

Waking Heart Rate _____

Standing Heart Rate _____

Waking Weight _____ Hours of Sleep _____

Quality of Sleep 1 2 3 4 5 6 7 8 9 10

Mood State 1 2 3 4 5 6 7 8 9 10

Goal _____

Workout _____

Specific Task _____

Actual Workout Time _____

Distance _____ Cadence _____

Average Heart Rate _____ Power _____

Interval 1: TIME _____ HR _____ P _____
Interval 2: TIME _____ HR _____ P _____
Interval 3: TIME _____ HR _____ P _____
Interval 4: TIME _____ HR _____ P _____
Interval 5: TIME _____ HR _____ P _____

Workout Notes _____

Personal Notes _____

Friday ■ Date: ___ / ___ / ___

Waking Heart Rate _____

Standing Heart Rate _____

Waking Weight _____ Hours of Sleep _____

Quality of Sleep 1 2 3 4 5 6 7 8 9 10

Mood State 1 2 3 4 5 6 7 8 9 10

Goal _____

Workout _____

Specific Task _____

Actual Workout Time _____

Distance _____ Cadence _____

Average Heart Rate _____ Power _____

Interval 1: TIME _____ HR _____ P _____
Interval 2: TIME _____ HR _____ P _____
Interval 3: TIME _____ HR _____ P _____
Interval 4: TIME _____ HR _____ P _____
Interval 5: TIME _____ HR _____ P _____

Workout Notes _____

Personal Notes _____

Saturday ■ Date: ___ / ___ / ___

Waking Heart Rate _____

Standing Heart Rate _____

Waking Weight _____ Hours of Sleep _____

Quality of Sleep 1 2 3 4 5 6 7 8 9 10

Mood State 1 2 3 4 5 6 7 8 9 10

Goal _____

Workout _____

Specific Task _____

Actual Workout Time _____

Distance _____ Cadence _____

Average Heart Rate _____ Power _____

Interval 1: TIME _____ HR _____ P _____
Interval 2: TIME _____ HR _____ P _____
Interval 3: TIME _____ HR _____ P _____
Interval 4: TIME _____ HR _____ P _____
Interval 5: TIME _____ HR _____ P _____

Workout Notes _____

Personal Notes _____

Week #

Sunday ■ Date: ___ / ___ / ___

Waking Heart Rate _____

Standing Heart Rate _____

Waking Weight _____ Hours of Sleep _____

Quality of Sleep 1 2 3 4 5 6 7 8 9 10

Mood State 1 2 3 4 5 6 7 8 9 10

Goal _____

Workout _____

Specific Task _____

Actual Workout Time _____

Distance _____ Cadence _____

Average Heart Rate _____ Power _____

Interval 1: TIME _____ HR _____ P _____

Interval 2: TIME _____ HR _____ P _____

Interval 3: TIME _____ HR _____ P _____

Interval 4: TIME _____ HR _____ P _____

Interval 5: TIME _____ HR _____ P _____

Workout Notes _____

Personal Notes _____

Weekly Summary

Hours of Cycling: _____ Year-to-Date: _____

Miles/Kilometers: _____ Year-to-Date: _____

Hours of Strength Training: _____ Year-to-Date: _____

Hours of Other Activities: _____

_____ Year-to-Date: _____

_____ Year-to-Date: _____

_____ Year-to-Date: _____

_____ Year-to-Date: _____

Total Training Hours: _____

Number of Workouts Planned: _____

Number of Workouts Completed: _____

Average Hours of Sleep: _____

Average Quality of Sleep: _____

Average Mood State: _____

Time Spent in Heart Rate/Power Ranges:

CTS RANGES	TIME	CTS RANGES	TIME	OTHER WORKOUTS	TIME
RecoveryMiles™	_____	SteadyState™	_____	_____	_____
FoundationMiles™	_____	ClimbingRepeats™	_____		
EnduranceMiles™	_____	Max Effort	_____		
Tempo™	_____				

Personal Notes: _____

Weekly Strength Training Record

Race Results

Race #1 _____ Date: ___/___/___

Time _____ Distance _____

Goal _____

Result _____

Average Heart Rate _____ Power _____

Food/Fluid Intake _____

Personal Notes _____

_____

_____

Race #2 _____ Date: ___/___/___

Time _____ Distance _____

Goal _____

Result _____

Average Heart Rate _____ Power _____

Food/Fluid Intake _____

Personal Notes _____

_____

_____

Exercise	Date:			Date:			Date:		
	SET 1 lbs./reps	SET 2 lbs./reps	SET 3 lbs./reps	SET 1 lbs./reps	SET 2 lbs./reps	SET 3 lbs./reps	SET 1 lbs./reps	SET 2 lbs./reps	SET 3 lbs./reps

Week # _____   Goal: _____

Monday ■ Date: ___/___/___

Waking Heart Rate _____

Standing Heart Rate _____

Waking Weight _____ Hours of Sleep _____

Quality of Sleep   1 2 3 4 5 6 7 8 9 10

Mood State   1 2 3 4 5 6 7 8 9 10

Goal _____

Workout _____

Specific Task _____

Actual Workout Time _____

Distance _____ Cadence _____ Power _____

Average Heart Rate _____

Interval 1: TIME _____ HR _____ P _____

Interval 2: TIME _____ HR _____ P _____

Interval 3: TIME _____ HR _____ P _____

Interval 4: TIME _____ HR _____ P _____

Interval 5: TIME _____ HR _____ P _____

Workout Notes _____

Personal Notes _____

Tuesday ■ Date: ___/___/___

Waking Heart Rate _____

Standing Heart Rate _____

Waking Weight _____ Hours of Sleep _____

Quality of Sleep   1 2 3 4 5 6 7 8 9 10

Mood State   1 2 3 4 5 6 7 8 9 10

Goal _____

Workout _____

Specific Task _____

Actual Workout Time _____

Distance _____ Cadence _____ Power _____

Average Heart Rate _____

Interval 1: TIME _____ HR _____ P _____

Interval 2: TIME _____ HR _____ P _____

Interval 3: TIME _____ HR _____ P _____

Interval 4: TIME _____ HR _____ P _____

Interval 5: TIME _____ HR _____ P _____

Workout Notes _____

Personal Notes _____

Wednesday ■ Date: ___/___/___

Waking Heart Rate _____

Standing Heart Rate _____

Waking Weight _____ Hours of Sleep _____

Quality of Sleep   1 2 3 4 5 6 7 8 9 10

Mood State   1 2 3 4 5 6 7 8 9 10

Goal _____

Workout _____

Specific Task _____

Actual Workout Time _____

Distance _____ Cadence _____ Power _____

Average Heart Rate _____

Interval 1: TIME _____ HR _____ P _____

Interval 2: TIME _____ HR _____ P _____

Interval 3: TIME _____ HR _____ P _____

Interval 4: TIME _____ HR _____ P _____

Interval 5: TIME _____ HR _____ P _____

Workout Notes _____

Personal Notes _____

Thursday ■ Date: ___ / ___ / ___

Waking Heart Rate ___

Standing Heart Rate ___

Waking Weight ___ Hours of Sleep ___

Quality of Sleep 1 2 3 4 5 6 7 8 9 10

Mood State 1 2 3 4 5 6 7 8 9 10

Goal ___

Workout ___

Specific Task ___

Actual Workout Time ___

Distance ___ Cadence ___

Average Heart Rate ___ Power ___

Interval 1: TIME ___ HR ___ P ___
Interval 2: TIME ___ HR ___ P ___
Interval 3: TIME ___ HR ___ P ___
Interval 4: TIME ___ HR ___ P ___
Interval 5: TIME ___ HR ___ P ___

Workout Notes ___

Personal Notes ___

Friday ■ Date: ___ / ___ / ___

Waking Heart Rate ___

Standing Heart Rate ___

Waking Weight ___ Hours of Sleep ___

Quality of Sleep 1 2 3 4 5 6 7 8 9 10

Mood State 1 2 3 4 5 6 7 8 9 10

Goal ___

Workout ___

Specific Task ___

Actual Workout Time ___

Distance ___ Cadence ___

Average Heart Rate ___ Power ___

Interval 1: TIME ___ HR ___ P ___
Interval 2: TIME ___ HR ___ P ___
Interval 3: TIME ___ HR ___ P ___
Interval 4: TIME ___ HR ___ P ___
Interval 5: TIME ___ HR ___ P ___

Workout Notes ___

Personal Notes ___

Saturday ■ Date: ___ / ___ / ___

Waking Heart Rate ___

Standing Heart Rate ___

Waking Weight ___ Hours of Sleep ___

Quality of Sleep 1 2 3 4 5 6 7 8 9 10

Mood State 1 2 3 4 5 6 7 8 9 10

Goal ___

Workout ___

Specific Task ___

Actual Workout Time ___

Distance ___ Cadence ___

Average Heart Rate ___ Power ___

Interval 1: TIME ___ HR ___ P ___
Interval 2: TIME ___ HR ___ P ___
Interval 3: TIME ___ HR ___ P ___
Interval 4: TIME ___ HR ___ P ___
Interval 5: TIME ___ HR ___ P ___

Workout Notes ___

Personal Notes ___

Sunday ■ Date: ___ / ___ / ___

Waking Heart Rate ___

Standing Heart Rate ___

Waking Weight ___ Hours of Sleep ___

Quality of Sleep 1 2 3 4 5 6 7 8 9 10

Mood State 1 2 3 4 5 6 7 8 9 10

Goal ___

Workout ___

Specific Task ___

Actual Workout Time ___

Distance ___ Cadence ___

Average Heart Rate ___ Power ___

Interval 1: TIME ___ HR ___ P ___

Interval 2: TIME ___ HR ___ P ___

Interval 3: TIME ___ HR ___ P ___

Interval 4: TIME ___ HR ___ P ___

Interval 5: TIME ___ HR ___ P ___

Workout Notes ___

Personal Notes ___

Weekly Summary

Hours of Cycling: ___ Year-to-Date: ___

Miles/Kilometers: ___ Year-to-Date: ___

Hours of Strength Training: ___ Year-to-Date: ___

Hours of Other Activities: ___

___ Year-to-Date: ___

___ Year-to-Date: ___

___ Year-to-Date: ___

___ Year-to-Date: ___

Total Training Hours: ___

Number of Workouts Planned: ___

Number of Workouts Completed: ___

Average Hours of Sleep: ___

Average Quality of Sleep: ___

Average Mood State: ___

Time Spent in Heart Rate/Power Ranges:

CTS RANGES	TIME	CTS RANGES	TIME	OTHER WORKOUTS	TIME
RecoveryMiles™		SteadyState™			
FoundationMiles™		ClimbingRepeats™			
EnduranceMiles™		Max Effort			
Tempo™					

Personal Notes: ___

Weekly Strength Training Record

Exercise	Date:			Date:			Date:		
	SET 1 lbs. / reps	SET 2 lbs. / reps	SET 3 lbs. / reps	SET 1 lbs. / reps	SET 2 lbs. / reps	SET 3 lbs. / reps	SET 1 lbs. / reps	SET 2 lbs. / reps	SET 3 lbs. / reps

Race Results

Race #1 Date: __/__/__

Time_____ Distance_____

Goal_____

Result_____

Average Heart Rate_____ Power_____

Food/Fluid Intake_____

Personal Notes_____

_____

_____

Race #2 Date: __/__/__

Time_____ Distance_____

Goal_____

Result_____

Average Heart Rate_____ Power_____

Food/Fluid Intake_____

Personal _____

Week # _____   Goal: _____

Monday ■ Date: ___ / ___ / ___

Waking Heart Rate _____

Standing Heart Rate _____

Waking Weight _____ Hours of Sleep _____

Quality of Sleep   1 2 3 4 5 6 7 8 9 10

Mood State   1 2 3 4 5 6 7 8 9 10

Goal _____

Workout _____

Specific Task _____

Actual Workout Time _____

Distance _____ Cadence _____

Average Heart Rate _____ Power _____

Interval 1: TIME _____ HR _____ P _____

Interval 2: TIME _____ HR _____ P _____

Interval 3: TIME _____ HR _____ P _____

Interval 4: TIME _____ HR _____ P _____

Interval 5: TIME _____ HR _____ P _____

Workout Notes _____

_____

Personal Notes _____

_____

Tuesday ■ Date: ___ / ___ / ___

Waking Heart Rate _____

Standing Heart Rate _____

Waking Weight _____ Hours of Sleep _____

Quality of Sleep   1 2 3 4 5 6 7 8 9 10

Mood State   1 2 3 4 5 6 7 8 9 10

Goal _____

Workout _____

Specific Task _____

Actual Workout Time _____

Distance _____ Cadence _____

Average Heart Rate _____ Power _____

Interval 1: TIME _____ HR _____ P _____

Interval 2: TIME _____ HR _____ P _____

Interval 3: TIME _____ HR _____ P _____

Interval 4: TIME _____ HR _____ P _____

Interval 5: TIME _____ HR _____ P _____

Workout Notes _____

_____

Personal Notes _____

_____

Wednesd[ay] ■ Date: ___ / ___ / ___

Waking Heart Rate _____

Standing Heart Rate _____

Waking Weight _____ Hours of Sleep _____

Quality of Sleep   1 2 3 4 5 6 7 8 9 10

Mood State   1 2 3 4 5 6 7 8 9 10

Goal _____

Workout _____

Specific Task _____

Actual Workout Time _____

Distance _____ Cadence _____

Average Heart Rate _____ Power _____

Interval 1: TIME _____ HR _____ P _____

Interval 2: TIME _____ HR _____ P _____

Interval 3: TIME _____ HR _____ P _____

Interval 4: TIME _____ HR _____ P _____

Interval 5: TIME _____ HR _____ P _____

Workout Notes _____

Personal Notes _____

Thursday ■ Date: ____ / ____ / ____

Waking Heart Rate _____

Standing Heart Rate _____

Waking Weight _____ Hours of Sleep _____

Quality of Sleep 1 2 3 4 5 6 7 8 9 10

Mood State 1 2 3 4 5 6 7 8 9 10

Goal _____

Workout _____

Specific Task _____

Actual Workout Time _____

Distance _____ Cadence _____

Average Heart Rate _____ Power _____

Interval 1:	TIME ____ HR ____	P ____
Interval 2:	TIME ____ HR ____	P ____
Interval 3:	TIME ____ HR ____	P ____
Interval 4:	TIME ____ HR ____	P ____
Interval 5:	TIME ____ HR ____	P ____

Workout Notes _____

Personal Notes _____

Friday ■ Date: ____ / ____ / ____

Waking Heart Rate _____

Standing Heart Rate _____

Waking Weight _____ Hours of Sleep _____

Quality of Sleep 1 2 3 4 5 6 7 8 9 10

Mood State 1 2 3 4 5 6 7 8 9 10

Goal _____

Workout _____

Specific Task _____

Actual Workout Time _____

Distance _____ Cadence _____

Average Heart Rate _____ Power _____

Interval 1:	TIME ____ HR ____	P ____
Interval 2:	TIME ____ HR ____	P ____
Interval 3:	TIME ____ HR ____	P ____
Interval 4:	TIME ____ HR ____	P ____
Interval 5:	TIME ____ HR ____	P ____

Workout Notes _____

Personal Notes _____

Saturday ■ Date: ____ / ____ / ____

Waking Heart Rate _____

Standing Heart Rate _____

Waking Weight _____ Hours of Sleep _____

Quality of Sleep 1 2 3 4 5 6 7 8 9 10

Mood State 1 2 3 4 5 6 7 8 9 10

Goal _____

Workout _____

Specific Task _____

Actual Workout Time _____

Distance _____ Cadence _____

Average Heart Rate _____ Power _____

Interval 1:	TIME ____ HR ____	P ____
Interval 2:	TIME ____ HR ____	P ____
Interval 3:	TIME ____ HR ____	P ____
Interval 4:	TIME ____ HR ____	P ____
Interval 5:	TIME ____ HR ____	P ____

Workout Notes _____

Personal Notes _____

Week #

Sunday ■ Date: ___ / ___ / ___

Waking Heart Rate ___

Standing Heart Rate ___

Waking Weight ___ Hours of Sleep ___

Quality of Sleep 1 2 3 4 5 6 7 8 9 10

Mood State 1 2 3 4 5 6 7 8 9 10

Goal ___

Workout ___

Specific Task ___

Actual Workout Time ___

Distance ___ Cadence ___

Average Heart Rate ___ Power ___

Interval 1: TIME ___ HR ___ P ___

Interval 2: TIME ___ HR ___ P ___

Interval 3: TIME ___ HR ___ P ___

Interval 4: TIME ___ HR ___ P ___

Interval 5: TIME ___ HR ___ P ___

Workout Notes ___

Personal Notes ___

Weekly Summary

Hours of Cycling: ___ Year-to-Date: ___

Miles/Kilometers: ___ Year-to-Date: ___

Hours of Strength Training: ___ Year-to-Date: ___

Hours of Other Activities: ___

___ Year-to-Date: ___

___ Year-to-Date: ___

___ Year-to-Date: ___

___ Year-to-Date: ___

Total Training Hours: ___

Number of Workouts Planned: ___

Number of Workouts Completed: ___

Average Hours of Sleep: ___

Average Quality of Sleep: ___

Average Mood State: ___

Time Spent in Heart Rate/Power Ranges:

CTS RANGES	TIME	CTS RANGES	TIME	OTHER WORKOUTS	TIME
RecoveryMiles™	___	SteadyState™	___		___
FoundationMiles™	___	ClimbingRepeats™	___		___
EnduranceMiles™	___	Max Effort	___		___
Tempo™	___				

Personal Notes: ___

Race Results

Race #1 _____ Date: ___/___/___

Time _____ Distance _____

Goal _____

Result _____

Average Heart Rate _____ Power _____

Food/Fluid Intake _____

Personal Notes _____

Race #2 _____ Date: ___/___/___

Time _____ Distance _____

Goal _____

Result _____

Average Heart Rate _____ Power _____

Food/Fluid Intake _____

Personal Notes _____

Week # [ ]   Weekly Strength Training Record

Exercise	Date:			Date:			Date:		
	SET 1 lbs. / reps	SET 2 lbs. / reps	SET 3 lbs. / reps	SET 1 lbs. / reps	SET 2 lbs. / reps	SET 3 lbs. / reps	SET 1 lbs. / reps	SET 2 lbs. / reps	SET 3 lbs. / reps

Week # _____   Goal: _____

Monday ■ Date: ___ / ___ / ___

Waking Heart Rate _____

Standing Heart Rate _____

Waking Weight _____ Hours of Sleep _____

Quality of Sleep 1 2 3 4 5 6 7 8 9 10

Mood State 1 2 3 4 5 6 7 8 9 10

Goal _____

Workout _____

Specific Task _____

Actual Workout Time _____

Distance _____ Cadence _____

Average Heart Rate _____ Power _____

Interval 1: TIME _____ HR _____ P _____

Interval 2: TIME _____ HR _____ P _____

Interval 3: TIME _____ HR _____ P _____

Interval 4: TIME _____ HR _____ P _____

Interval 5: TIME _____ HR _____ P _____

Workout Notes _____

Personal Notes _____

Tuesday ■ Date: ___ / ___ / ___

Waking Heart Rate _____

Standing Heart Rate _____

Waking Weight _____ Hours of Sleep _____

Quality of Sleep 1 2 3 4 5 6 7 8 9 10

Mood State 1 2 3 4 5 6 7 8 9 10

Goal _____

Workout _____

Specific Task _____

Actual Workout Time _____

Distance _____ Cadence _____

Average Heart Rate _____ Power _____

Interval 1: TIME _____ HR _____ P _____

Interval 2: TIME _____ HR _____ P _____

Interval 3: TIME _____ HR _____ P _____

Interval 4: TIME _____ HR _____ P _____

Interval 5: TIME _____ HR _____ P _____

Workout Notes _____

Personal Notes _____

Wednesday ■ Date: ___ / ___ / ___

Waking Heart Rate _____

Standing Heart Rate _____

Waking Weight _____ Hours of Sleep _____

Quality of Sleep 1 2 3 4 5 6 7 8 9 10

Mood State 1 2 3 4 5 6 7 8 9 10

Goal _____

Workout _____

Specific Task _____

Actual Workout Time _____

Distance _____ Cadence _____

Average Heart Rate _____ Power _____

Interval 1: TIME _____ HR _____ P _____

Interval 2: TIME _____ HR _____ P _____

Interval 3: TIME _____ HR _____ P _____

Interval 4: TIME _____ HR _____ P _____

Interval 5: TIME _____ HR _____ P _____

Workout Notes _____

Personal Notes _____

Thursday ▪ Date: ____ / ____ / ____

Waking Heart Rate _____

Standing Heart Rate _____

Waking Weight _____ Hours of Sleep _____

Quality of Sleep 1 2 3 4 5 6 7 8 9 10

Mood State 1 2 3 4 5 6 7 8 9 10

Goal _____

Workout _____

Specific Task _____

Actual Workout Time _____

Distance _____ Cadence _____ Power _____

Average Heart Rate _____

Interval 1:	TIME _____	HR _____	P _____
Interval 2:	TIME _____	HR _____	P _____
Interval 3:	TIME _____	HR _____	P _____
Interval 4:	TIME _____	HR _____	P _____
Interval 5:	TIME _____	HR _____	P _____

Workout Notes _____

Personal Notes _____

Friday ▪ Date: ____ / ____ / ____

Waking Heart Rate _____

Standing Heart Rate _____

Waking Weight _____ Hours of Sleep _____

Quality of Sleep 1 2 3 4 5 6 7 8 9 10

Mood State 1 2 3 4 5 6 7 8 9 10

Goal _____

Workout _____

Specific Task _____

Actual Workout Time _____

Distance _____ Cadence _____ Power _____

Average Heart Rate _____

Interval 1:	TIME _____	HR _____	P _____
Interval 2:	TIME _____	HR _____	P _____
Interval 3:	TIME _____	HR _____	P _____
Interval 4:	TIME _____	HR _____	P _____
Interval 5:	TIME _____	HR _____	P _____

Workout Notes _____

Personal Notes _____

Saturday ▪ Date: ____ / ____ / ____

Waking Heart Rate _____

Standing Heart Rate _____

Waking Weight _____ Hours of Sleep _____

Quality of Sleep 1 2 3 4 5 6 7 8 9 10

Mood State 1 2 3 4 5 6 7 8 9 10

Goal _____

Workout _____

Specific Task _____

Actual Workout Time _____

Distance _____ Cadence _____ Power _____

Average Heart Rate _____

Interval 1:	TIME _____	HR _____	P _____
Interval 2:	TIME _____	HR _____	P _____
Interval 3:	TIME _____	HR _____	P _____
Interval 4:	TIME _____	HR _____	P _____
Interval 5:	TIME _____	HR _____	P _____

Workout Notes _____

Personal Notes _____

Week # ____

Sunday ■ Date: ____ / ____ / ____

Waking Heart Rate _____

Standing Heart Rate _____

Waking Weight _____ Hours of Sleep _____

Quality of Sleep 1 2 3 4 5 6 7 8 9 10

_____

Mood State 1 2 3 4 5 6 7 8 9 10

_____

Goal _____

Workout _____

Specific Task _____

Actual Workout Time _____

Distance _____ Cadence _____

Average Heart Rate _____ Power _____

Interval 1: TIME _____ HR _____ P _____

Interval 2: TIME _____ HR _____ P _____

Interval 3: TIME _____ HR _____ P _____

Interval 4: TIME _____ HR _____ P _____

Interval 5: TIME _____ HR _____ P _____

Workout Notes _____

Personal Notes _____

Weekly Summary

Hours of Cycling: _____ Year-to-Date: _____

Miles/Kilometers: _____ Year-to-Date: _____

Hours of Strength Training: _____ Year-to-Date: _____

Hours of Other Activities: _____

_____ Year-to-Date: _____

_____ Year-to-Date: _____

_____ Year-to-Date: _____

_____ Year-to-Date: _____

Total Training Hours: _____

Number of Workouts Planned: _____

Number of Workouts Completed: _____

Average Hours of Sleep: _____

Average Quality of Sleep: _____

Average Mood State: _____

Time Spent in Heart Rate/Power Ranges:

CTS RANGES	TIME	CTS RANGES	TIME	OTHER WORKOUTS	TIME
RecoveryMiles™		SteadyState™			
FoundationMiles™		ClimbingRepeats™			
EnduranceMiles™		Max Effort			
Tempo™					

Personal Notes: _____

Weekly Strength Training Record

Exercise	Date:			Date:			Date:		
	SET 1 lbs. / reps	SET 2 lbs. / reps	SET 3 lbs. / reps	SET 1 lbs. / reps	SET 2 lbs. / reps	SET 3 lbs. / reps	SET 1 lbs. / reps	SET 2 lbs. / reps	SET 3 lbs. / reps

Race Results

Race #1 _____ Date: ___/___/___

Time_____ Distance_____

Goal_____

Result_____

Average Heart Rate _____ Power_____

Food/Fluid Intake_____

Personal Notes_____

_____

_____

Race #2 _____ Date: ___/___/___

Time_____ Distance_____

Goal_____

Result_____

Average Heart Rate _____ Power_____

Food/Fluid Intake_____

Personal Notes_____

_____

_____

Week # _____   Goal: _____

Monday ■ Date: ___ / ___ / ___

Waking Heart Rate _____

Standing Heart Rate _____

Waking Weight _____ Hours of Sleep _____

Quality of Sleep 1 2 3 4 5 6 7 8 9 10

Mood State 1 2 3 4 5 6 7 8 9 10

Goal _____

Workout _____

Specific Task _____

Actual Workout Time _____

Distance _____ Cadence _____

Average Heart Rate _____ Power _____

Interval 1: TIME _____ HR _____ P _____
Interval 2: TIME _____ HR _____ P _____
Interval 3: TIME _____ HR _____ P _____
Interval 4: TIME _____ HR _____ P _____
Interval 5: TIME _____ HR _____ P _____

Workout Notes _____

Personal Notes _____

Tuesday ■ Date: ___ / ___ / ___

Waking Heart Rate _____

Standing Heart Rate _____

Waking Weight _____ Hours of Sleep _____

Quality of Sleep 1 2 3 4 5 6 7 8 9 10

Mood State 1 2 3 4 5 6 7 8 9 10

Goal _____

Workout _____

Specific Task _____

Actual Workout Time _____

Distance _____ Cadence _____

Average Heart Rate _____ Power _____

Interval 1: TIME _____ HR _____ P _____
Interval 2: TIME _____ HR _____ P _____
Interval 3: TIME _____ HR _____ P _____
Interval 4: TIME _____ HR _____ P _____
Interval 5: TIME _____ HR _____ P _____

Workout Notes _____

Personal Notes _____

Wednesday ■ Date: ___ / ___ / ___

Waking Heart Rate _____

Standing Heart Rate _____

Waking Weight _____ Hours of Sleep _____

Quality of Sleep 1 2 3 4 5 6 7 8 9 10

Mood State 1 2 3 4 5 6 7 8 9 10

Goal _____

Workout _____

Specific Task _____

Actual Workout Time _____

Distance _____ Cadence _____

Average Heart Rate _____ Power _____

Interval 1: TIME _____ HR _____ P _____
Interval 2: TIME _____ HR _____ P _____
Interval 3: TIME _____ HR _____ P _____
Interval 4: TIME _____ HR _____ P _____
Interval 5: TIME _____ HR _____ P _____

Workout Notes _____

Personal Notes _____

Thursday ■ Date: ___ / ___ / ___

Waking Heart Rate _____

Standing Heart Rate _____

Waking Weight _____ Hours of Sleep _____

Quality of Sleep 1 2 3 4 5 6 7 8 9 10

Mood State 1 2 3 4 5 6 7 8 9 10

Goal _____

Workout _____

Specific Task _____

Actual Workout Time _____

Distance _____ Cadence _____ Power _____

Average Heart Rate _____

Interval 1:	TIME _____ HR _____	P _____
Interval 2:	TIME _____ HR _____	P _____
Interval 3:	TIME _____ HR _____	P _____
Interval 4:	TIME _____ HR _____	P _____
Interval 5:	TIME _____ HR _____	P _____

Workout Notes _____

Personal Notes _____

Friday ■ Date: ___ / ___ / ___

Waking Heart Rate _____

Standing Heart Rate _____

Waking Weight _____ Hours of Sleep _____

Quality of Sleep 1 2 3 4 5 6 7 8 9 10

Mood State 1 2 3 4 5 6 7 8 9 10

Goal _____

Workout _____

Specific Task _____

Actual Workout Time _____

Distance _____ Cadence _____ Power _____

Average Heart Rate _____

Interval 1:	TIME _____ HR _____	P _____
Interval 2:	TIME _____ HR _____	P _____
Interval 3:	TIME _____ HR _____	P _____
Interval 4:	TIME _____ HR _____	P _____
Interval 5:	TIME _____ HR _____	P _____

Workout Notes _____

Personal Notes _____

Saturday ■ Date: ___ / ___ / ___

Waking Heart Rate _____

Standing Heart Rate _____

Waking Weight _____ Hours of Sleep _____

Quality of Sleep 1 2 3 4 5 6 7 8 9 10

Mood State 1 2 3 4 5 6 7 8 9 10

Goal _____

Workout _____

Specific Task _____

Actual Workout Time _____

Distance _____ Cadence _____ Power _____

Average Heart Rate _____

Interval 1:	TIME _____ HR _____	P _____
Interval 2:	TIME _____ HR _____	P _____
Interval 3:	TIME _____ HR _____	P _____
Interval 4:	TIME _____ HR _____	P _____
Interval 5:	TIME _____ HR _____	P _____

Workout Notes _____

Personal Notes _____

Week # _____

Sunday ■ Date: ____ / ____ / ____

Waking Heart Rate _____

Standing Heart Rate _____

Waking Weight _____ Hours of Sleep _____

Quality of Sleep 1 2 3 4 5 6 7 8 9 10

Mood State 1 2 3 4 5 6 7 8 9 10

Goal _____

Workout _____

Specific Task _____

Actual Workout Time _____

Distance _____ Cadence _____

Average Heart Rate _____ Power _____

Interval 1:	TIME _____	HR _____	P _____
Interval 2:	TIME _____	HR _____	P _____
Interval 3:	TIME _____	HR _____	P _____
Interval 4:	TIME _____	HR _____	P _____
Interval 5:	TIME _____	HR _____	P _____

Workout Notes _____

Personal Notes _____

Weekly Summary

Hours of Cycling: _____ Year-to-Date: _____

Miles/Kilometers: _____ Year-to-Date: _____

Hours of Strength Training: _____ Year-to-Date: _____

Hours of Other Activities: _____

_____ Year-to-Date: _____

_____ Year-to-Date: _____

_____ Year-to-Date: _____

Total Training Hours: _____ Year-to-Date: _____

Number of Workouts Planned: _____

Number of Workouts Completed: _____

Average Hours of Sleep: _____

Average Quality of Sleep: _____

Average Mood State: _____

Time Spent in Heart Rate/Power Ranges:

CTS RANGES	TIME	CTS RANGES	TIME	OTHER WORKOUTS	TIME
RecoveryMiles™	_____	SteadyState™	_____		_____
FoundationMiles™	_____	ClimbingRepeats™	_____		_____
EnduranceMiles™	_____	Max Effort	_____		_____
Tempo™	_____				

Personal Notes: _____

Weekly Strength Training Record

Race Results

Exercise	Date:						Date:						Date:					
	SET 1		SET 2		SET 3		SET 1		SET 2		SET 3		SET 1		SET 2		SET 3	
	lbs.	reps	lbs.	reps	lbs.	reps	lbs.	reps	lbs.	reps	lbs.	reps	lbs.	reps	lbs.	reps	lbs.	reps

Race #1 _____ Date: ___ / ___ / ___

Time _____ Distance _____

Goal _____

Result _____

Average Heart Rate _____ Power _____

Food/Fluid Intake _____

Personal Notes _____

_____

_____

Race #2 _____ Date: ___ / ___ / ___

Time _____ Distance _____

Goal _____

Result _____

Average Heart Rate _____ Power _____

Food/Fluid Intake _____

Personal Notes _____

_____

_____

Week # _____ Goal: _____

Monday ■ Date: ___ / ___ / ___

Waking Heart Rate _____

Standing Heart Rate _____

Waking Weight _____ Hours of Sleep _____

Quality of Sleep 1 2 3 4 5 6 7 8 9 10

Mood State 1 2 3 4 5 6 7 8 9 10

Goal _____

Workout _____

Specific Task _____

Actual Workout Time _____

Distance _____ Cadence _____

Average Heart Rate _____ Power _____

Interval 1: TIME _____ HR _____ P _____

Interval 2: TIME _____ HR _____ P _____

Interval 3: TIME _____ HR _____ P _____

Interval 4: TIME _____ HR _____ P _____

Interval 5: TIME _____ HR _____ P _____

Workout Notes _____

Personal Notes _____

Tuesday ■ Date: ___ / ___ / ___

Waking Heart Rate _____

Standing Heart Rate _____

Waking Weight _____ Hours of Sleep _____

Quality of Sleep 1 2 3 4 5 6 7 8 9 10

Mood State 1 2 3 4 5 6 7 8 9 10

Goal _____

Workout _____

Specific Task _____

Actual Workout Time _____

Distance _____ Cadence _____

Average Heart Rate _____ Power _____

Interval 1: TIME _____ HR _____ P _____

Interval 2: TIME _____ HR _____ P _____

Interval 3: TIME _____ HR _____ P _____

Interval 4: TIME _____ HR _____ P _____

Interval 5: TIME _____ HR _____ P _____

Workout Notes _____

Personal Notes _____

Wednesday ■ Date: ___ / ___ / ___

Waking Heart Rate _____

Standing Heart Rate _____

Waking Weight _____ Hours of Sleep _____

Quality of Sleep 1 2 3 4 5 6 7 8 9 10

Mood State 1 2 3 4 5 6 7 8 9 10

Goal _____

Workout _____

Specific Task _____

Actual Workout Time _____

Distance _____ Cadence _____

Average Heart Rate _____ Power _____

Interval 1: TIME _____ HR _____ P _____

Interval 2: TIME _____ HR _____ P _____

Interval 3: TIME _____ HR _____ P _____

Interval 4: TIME _____ HR _____ P _____

Interval 5: TIME _____ HR _____ P _____

Workout Notes _____

Personal Notes _____

Thursday ■ Date: ___ / ___ / ___

Waking Heart Rate _____

Standing Heart Rate _____

Waking Weight _____ Hours of Sleep _____

Quality of Sleep 1 2 3 4 5 6 7 8 9 10

Mood State 1 2 3 4 5 6 7 8 9 10

Goal _____

Workout _____

Specific Task _____

Actual Workout Time _____

Distance _____ Cadence _____

Average Heart Rate _____ Power _____

Interval 1:	TIME _____	HR _____	P _____
Interval 2:	TIME _____	HR _____	P _____
Interval 3:	TIME _____	HR _____	P _____
Interval 4:	TIME _____	HR _____	P _____
Interval 5:	TIME _____	HR _____	P _____

Workout Notes _____

Personal Notes _____

Friday ■ Date: ___ / ___ / ___

Waking Heart Rate _____

Standing Heart Rate _____

Waking Weight _____ Hours of Sleep _____

Quality of Sleep 1 2 3 4 5 6 7 8 9 10

Mood State 1 2 3 4 5 6 7 8 9 10

Goal _____

Workout _____

Specific Task _____

Actual Workout Time _____

Distance _____ Cadence _____

Average Heart Rate _____ Power _____

Interval 1:	TIME _____	HR _____	P _____
Interval 2:	TIME _____	HR _____	P _____
Interval 3:	TIME _____	HR _____	P _____
Interval 4:	TIME _____	HR _____	P _____
Interval 5:	TIME _____	HR _____	P _____

Workout Notes _____

Personal Notes _____

Saturday ■ Date: ___ / ___ / ___

Waking Heart Rate _____

Standing Heart Rate _____

Waking Weight _____ Hours of Sleep _____

Quality of Sleep 1 2 3 4 5 6 7 8 9 10

Mood State 1 2 3 4 5 6 7 8 9 10

Goal _____

Workout _____

Specific Task _____

Actual Workout Time _____

Distance _____ Cadence _____

Average Heart Rate _____ Power _____

Interval 1:	TIME _____	HR _____	P _____
Interval 2:	TIME _____	HR _____	P _____
Interval 3:	TIME _____	HR _____	P _____
Interval 4:	TIME _____	HR _____	P _____
Interval 5:	TIME _____	HR _____	P _____

Workout Notes _____

Personal Notes _____

Sunday ■ Date: ____ / ____ / ____

Waking Heart Rate _____

Standing Heart Rate _____

Waking Weight _____ Hours of Sleep _____

Quality of Sleep   1 2 3 4 5 6 7 8 9 10

Mood State   1 2 3 4 5 6 7 8 9 10

Goal _____

Workout _____

Specific Task _____

Actual Workout Time _____

Distance _____ Cadence _____

Average Heart Rate _____ Power _____

Interval 1: TIME _____ HR _____ P _____

Interval 2: TIME _____ HR _____ P _____

Interval 3: TIME _____ HR _____ P _____

Interval 4: TIME _____ HR _____ P _____

Interval 5: TIME _____ HR _____ P _____

Workout Notes _____

_____

Personal Notes _____

_____

_____

Weekly Summary

Hours of Cycling: _____ Year-to-Date: _____

Miles/Kilometers: _____ Year-to-Date: _____

Hours of Strength Training: _____ Year-to-Date: _____

Hours of Other Activities: _____ Year-to-Date: _____

_____ Year-to-Date: _____

_____ Year-to-Date: _____

_____ Year-to-Date: _____

_____ Year-to-Date: _____

Total Training Hours: _____

Number of Workouts Planned: _____

Number of Workouts Completed: _____

Average Hours of Sleep: _____

Average Quality of Sleep: _____

Average Mood State: _____

Time Spent in Heart Rate/Power Ranges:

CTS RANGES	TIME	CTS RANGES	TIME	OTHER WORKOUTS	TIME
RecoveryMiles™		SteadyState™			
FoundationMiles™		ClimbingRepeats™			
EnduranceMiles™		Max Effort			
Tempo™					

Personal Notes: _____

_____

_____

Weekly Strength Training Record

Exercise	Date:						Date:						Date:					
	SET 1		SET 2		SET 3		SET 1		SET 2		SET 3		SET 1		SET 2		SET 3	
	lbs.	reps	lbs.	reps	lbs.	reps	lbs.	reps	lbs.	reps	lbs.	reps	lbs.	reps	lbs.	reps	lbs.	reps

Race Results

Race #1 _____ Date: ___ / ___ / ___

Time _____ Distance _____

Goal _____

Result _____

Average Heart Rate _____ Power _____

Food/Fluid Intake _____

Personal Notes _____

_____

_____

Race #2 _____ Date: ___ / ___ / ___

Time _____ Distance _____

Goal _____

Result _____

Average Heart Rate _____ Power _____

Food/Fluid Intake _____

Personal Notes _____

_____

_____

Monday ■ Date: ___ / ___ / ___

Waking Heart Rate _____

Standing Heart Rate _____

Waking Weight _____ Hours of Sleep _____

Quality of Sleep   1 2 3 4 5 6 7 8 9 10

Mood State   1 2 3 4 5 6 7 8 9 10

Goal _____

Workout _____

Specific Task _____

Actual Workout Time _____

Distance _____ Cadence _____

Average Heart Rate _____ Power _____

Interval 1: TIME _____ HR _____ P _____

Interval 2: TIME _____ HR _____ P _____

Interval 3: TIME _____ HR _____ P _____

Interval 4: TIME _____ HR _____ P _____

Interval 5: TIME _____ HR _____ P _____

Workout Notes _____

_____

Personal Notes _____

_____

Tuesday ■ Date: ___ / ___ / ___

Waking Heart Rate _____

Standing Heart Rate _____

Waking Weight _____ Hours of Sleep _____

Quality of Sleep   1 2 3 4 5 6 7 8 9 10

Mood State   1 2 3 4 5 6 7 8 9 10

Goal _____

Workout _____

Specific Task _____

Actual Workout Time _____

Distance _____ Cadence _____

Average Heart Rate _____ Power _____

Interval 1: TIME _____ HR _____ P _____

Interval 2: TIME _____ HR _____ P _____

Interval 3: TIME _____ HR _____ P _____

Interval 4: TIME _____ HR _____ P _____

Interval 5: TIME _____ HR _____ P _____

Workout Notes _____

_____

Personal Notes _____

_____

Wednesday ■ Date: ___ / ___ / ___

Waking Heart Rate _____

Standing Heart Rate _____

Waking Weight _____ Hours of Sleep _____

Quality of Sleep   1 2 3 4 5 6 7 8 9 10

Mood State   1 2 3 4 5 6 7 8 9 10

Goal _____

Workout _____

Specific Task _____

Actual Workout Time _____

Distance _____ Cadence _____

Average Heart Rate _____ Power _____

Interval 1: TIME _____ HR _____ P _____

Interval 2: TIME _____ HR _____ P _____

Interval 3: TIME _____ HR _____ P _____

Interval 4: TIME _____ HR _____ P _____

Interval 5: TIME _____ HR _____ P _____

Workout Notes _____

_____

Personal Notes _____

_____

Thursday ■ Date: ___ / ___ / ___

Waking Heart Rate _____

Standing Heart Rate _____

Waking Weight _____ Hours of Sleep _____

Quality of Sleep   1 2 3 4 5 6 7 8 9 10

Mood State   1 2 3 4 5 6 7 8 9 10

Goal _____

Workout _____

Specific Task _____

Actual Workout Time _____

Distance _____ Cadence _____

Average Heart Rate _____ Power _____

Interval 1: TIME _____ HR _____ P _____

Interval 2: TIME _____ HR _____ P _____

Interval 3: TIME _____ HR _____ P _____

Interval 4: TIME _____ HR _____ P _____

Interval 5: TIME _____ HR _____ P _____

Workout Notes _____

Personal Notes _____

Friday ■ Date: ___ / ___ / ___

Waking Heart Rate _____

Standing Heart Rate _____

Waking Weight _____ Hours of Sleep _____

Quality of Sleep   1 2 3 4 5 6 7 8 9 10

Mood State   1 2 3 4 5 6 7 8 9 10

Goal _____

Workout _____

Specific Task _____

Actual Workout Time _____

Distance _____ Cadence _____

Average Heart Rate _____ Power _____

Interval 1: TIME _____ HR _____ P _____

Interval 2: TIME _____ HR _____ P _____

Interval 3: TIME _____ HR _____ P _____

Interval 4: TIME _____ HR _____ P _____

Interval 5: TIME _____ HR _____ P _____

Workout Notes _____

Personal Notes _____

Saturday ■ Date: ___ / ___ / ___

Waking Heart Rate _____

Standing Heart Rate _____

Waking Weight _____ Hours of Sleep _____

Quality of Sleep   1 2 3 4 5 6 7 8 9 10

Mood State   1 2 3 4 5 6 7 8 9 10

Goal _____

Workout _____

Specific Task _____

Actual Workout Time _____

Distance _____ Cadence _____

Average Heart Rate _____ Power _____

Interval 1: TIME _____ HR _____ P _____

Interval 2: TIME _____ HR _____ P _____

Interval 3: TIME _____ HR _____ P _____

Interval 4: TIME _____ HR _____ P _____

Interval 5: TIME _____ HR _____ P _____

Workout Notes _____

Personal Notes _____

Week #

Sunday ■ Date: ___ / ___ / ___

Waking Heart Rate _____

Standing Heart Rate _____

Waking Weight _____ Hours of Sleep _____

Quality of Sleep 1 2 3 4 5 6 7 8 9 10

Mood State 1 2 3 4 5 6 7 8 9 10

Goal _____

Workout _____

Specific Task _____

Actual Workout Time _____

Distance _____ Cadence _____

Average Heart Rate _____ Power _____

Interval 1: TIME _____ HR _____ P _____
Interval 2: TIME _____ HR _____ P _____
Interval 3: TIME _____ HR _____ P _____
Interval 4: TIME _____ HR _____ P _____
Interval 5: TIME _____ HR _____ P _____

Workout Notes _____

Personal Notes _____

Weekly Summary

Hours of Cycling: _____ Year-to-Date: _____

Miles/Kilometers: _____ Year-to-Date: _____

Hours of Strength Training: _____ Year-to-Date: _____

Hours of Other Activities: _____

Year-to-Date: _____
Year-to-Date: _____
Year-to-Date: _____
Year-to-Date: _____

Total Training Hours: _____

Number of Workouts Planned: _____

Number of Workouts Completed: _____

Average Hours of Sleep: _____

Average Quality of Sleep: _____

Average Mood State: _____

Time Spent in Heart Rate/Power Ranges:

CTS RANGES	TIME	CTS RANGES	TIME	OTHER WORKOUTS	TIME
RecoveryMiles™	_____	SteadyState™	_____		_____
FoundationMiles™	_____	ClimbingRepeats™	_____		_____
EnduranceMiles™	_____	Max Effort	_____		_____
Tempo™	_____				

Personal Notes: _____

Weekly Strength Training Record

Exercise	Date:						Date:					
	SET 1		SET 2		SET 3		SET 1		SET 2		SET 3	
	lbs.	reps	lbs.	reps	lbs.	reps	lbs.	reps	lbs.	reps	lbs.	reps

Race Results

Race #1 _____ Date: ___/___/___

Time _____ Distance _____

Goal _____

Result _____

Average Heart Rate _____ Power _____

Food/Fluid Intake _____

Personal Notes _____

_____

Race #2 _____ Date: ___/___/___

Time _____ Distance _____

Goal _____

Result _____

Average Heart Rate _____ Power _____

Food/Fluid Intake _____

Personal Notes _____

_____

Monday ■ Date: ___ / ___ / ___

Waking Heart Rate ___
Standing Heart Rate ___
Waking Weight ___ Hours of Sleep ___
Quality of Sleep   1 2 3 4 5 6 7 8 9 10

Mood State   1 2 3 4 5 6 7 8 9 10

Goal ___
Workout ___
Specific Task ___
Actual Workout Time ___
Distance ___ Cadence ___ Power ___
Average Heart Rate ___

Interval 1: TIME ___ HR ___ P ___
Interval 2: TIME ___ HR ___ P ___
Interval 3: TIME ___ HR ___ P ___
Interval 4: TIME ___ HR ___ P ___
Interval 5: TIME ___ HR ___ P ___
Workout Notes ___

Personal Notes ___

Tuesday ■ Date: ___ / ___ / ___

Waking Heart Rate ___
Standing Heart Rate ___
Waking Weight ___ Hours of Sleep ___
Quality of Sleep   1 2 3 4 5 6 7 8 9 10

Mood State   1 2 3 4 5 6 7 8 9 10

Goal ___
Workout ___
Specific Task ___
Actual Workout Time ___
Distance ___ Cadence ___ Power ___
Average Heart Rate ___

Interval 1: TIME ___ HR ___ P ___
Interval 2: TIME ___ HR ___ P ___
Interval 3: TIME ___ HR ___ P ___
Interval 4: TIME ___ HR ___ P ___
Interval 5: TIME ___ HR ___ P ___
Workout Notes ___

Personal Notes ___

Wednesday ■ Date: ___ / ___ / ___

Waking Heart Rate ___
Standing Heart Rate ___
Waking Weight ___ Hours of Sleep ___
Quality of Sleep   1 2 3 4 5 6 7 8 9 10

Mood State   1 2 3 4 5 6 7 8 9 10

Goal ___
Workout ___
Specific Task ___
Actual Workout Time ___
Distance ___ Cadence ___ Power ___
Average Heart Rate ___

Interval 1: TIME ___ HR ___ P ___
Interval 2: TIME ___ HR ___ P ___
Interval 3: TIME ___ HR ___ P ___
Interval 4: TIME ___ HR ___ P ___
Interval 5: TIME ___ HR ___ P ___
Workout Notes ___

Personal Notes ___

Week #

Thursday ■ Date: ___ / ___ / ___

Waking Heart Rate _____

Standing Heart Rate _____

Waking Weight _____ Hours of Sleep _____

Quality of Sleep 1 2 3 4 5 6 7 8 9 10

Mood State 1 2 3 4 5 6 7 8 9 10

Goal _____

Workout _____

Specific Task _____

Actual Workout Time _____

Distance _____ Cadence _____

Average Heart Rate _____ Power _____

Interval 1: TIME _____ HR _____ P _____
Interval 2: TIME _____ HR _____ P _____
Interval 3: TIME _____ HR _____ P _____
Interval 4: TIME _____ HR _____ P _____
Interval 5: TIME _____ HR _____ P _____

Workout Notes _____

Personal Notes _____

Friday ■ Date: ___ / ___ / ___

Waking Heart Rate _____

Standing Heart Rate _____

Waking Weight _____ Hours of Sleep _____

Quality of Sleep 1 2 3 4 5 6 7 8 9 10

Mood State 1 2 3 4 5 6 7 8 9 10

Goal _____

Workout _____

Specific Task _____

Actual Workout Time _____

Distance _____ Cadence _____

Average Heart Rate _____ Power _____

Interval 1: TIME _____ HR _____ P _____
Interval 2: TIME _____ HR _____ P _____
Interval 3: TIME _____ HR _____ P _____
Interval 4: TIME _____ HR _____ P _____
Interval 5: TIME _____ HR _____ P _____

Workout Notes _____

Personal Notes _____

Saturday ■ Date: ___ / ___ / ___

Waking Heart Rate _____

Standing Heart Rate _____

Waking Weight _____ Hours of Sleep _____

Quality of Sleep 1 2 3 4 5 6 7 8 9 10

Mood State 1 2 3 4 5 6 7 8 9 10

Goal _____

Workout _____

Specific Task _____

Actual Workout Time _____

Distance _____ Cadence _____

Average Heart Rate _____ Power _____

Interval 1: TIME _____ HR _____ P _____
Interval 2: TIME _____ HR _____ P _____
Interval 3: TIME _____ HR _____ P _____
Interval 4: TIME _____ HR _____ P _____
Interval 5: TIME _____ HR _____ P _____

Workout Notes _____

Personal Notes _____

Sunday ■ Date: ___ / ___ / ___

Waking Heart Rate _____

Standing Heart Rate _____

Waking Weight _____ Hours of Sleep _____

Quality of Sleep 1 2 3 4 5 6 7 8 9 10

Mood State 1 2 3 4 5 6 7 8 9 10

Goal _____

Workout _____

Specific Task _____

Actual Workout Time _____

Distance _____ Cadence _____

Average Heart Rate _____ Power _____

Interval 1: TIME _____ HR _____ P _____
Interval 2: TIME _____ HR _____ P _____
Interval 3: TIME _____ HR _____ P _____
Interval 4: TIME _____ HR _____ P _____
Interval 5: TIME _____ HR _____ P _____

Workout Notes _____

Personal Notes _____

Weekly Summary

Hours of Cycling: _____ Year-to-Date: _____

Miles/Kilometers: _____ Year-to-Date: _____

Hours of Strength Training: _____ Year-to-Date: _____

Hours of Other Activities: _____ Year-to-Date: _____

_____ Year-to-Date: _____

_____ Year-to-Date: _____

_____ Year-to-Date: _____

Total Training Hours: _____

Number of Workouts Planned: _____

Number of Workouts Completed: _____

Average Hours of Sleep: _____

Average Quality of Sleep: _____

Average Mood State: _____

Time Spent in Heart Rate/Power Ranges:

CTS RANGES	TIME	CTS RANGES	TIME	OTHER WORKOUTS	TIME
RecoveryMiles™		SteadyState™			
FoundationMiles™		ClimbingRepeats™			
EnduranceMiles™		Max Effort			
Tempo™					

Personal Notes: _____

Weekly Strength Training Record

Exercise	Date:						Date:						Date:					
	SET 1		SET 2		SET 3		SET 1		SET 2		SET 3		SET 1		SET 2		SET 3	
	lbs.	reps	lbs.	reps	lbs.	reps	lbs.	reps	lbs.	reps	lbs.	reps	lbs.	reps	lbs.	reps	lbs.	reps

Race Results

Race #1 _____ Date: __ / __ / __

Time _____ Distance _____

Goal _____

Result _____

Average Heart Rate _____ Power _____

Food/Fluid Intake _____

Personal Notes _____

_____

_____

Race #2 _____ Date: __ / __ / __

Time _____ Distance _____

Goal _____

Result _____

Average Heart Rate _____ Power _____

Food/Fluid Intake _____

Personal Notes _____

_____

_____

Week # _____   Goal: _____

Monday ■ Date: ___ / ___ / ___

Waking Heart Rate _____

Standing Heart Rate _____

Waking Weight _____ Hours of Sleep _____

Quality of Sleep 1 2 3 4 5 6 7 8 9 10

Mood State 1 2 3 4 5 6 7 8 9 10

Goal _____

Workout _____

Specific Task _____

Actual Workout Time _____

Distance _____ Cadence _____

Average Heart Rate _____ Power _____

Interval 1: TIME _____ HR _____ P _____
Interval 2: TIME _____ HR _____ P _____
Interval 3: TIME _____ HR _____ P _____
Interval 4: TIME _____ HR _____ P _____
Interval 5: TIME _____ HR _____ P _____

Workout Notes _____

Personal Notes _____

Tuesday ■ Date: ___ / ___ / ___

Waking Heart Rate _____

Standing Heart Rate _____

Waking Weight _____ Hours of Sleep _____

Quality of Sleep 1 2 3 4 5 6 7 8 9 10

Mood State 1 2 3 4 5 6 7 8 9 10

Goal _____

Workout _____

Specific Task _____

Actual Workout Time _____

Distance _____ Cadence _____

Average Heart Rate _____ Power _____

Interval 1: TIME _____ HR _____ P _____
Interval 2: TIME _____ HR _____ P _____
Interval 3: TIME _____ HR _____ P _____
Interval 4: TIME _____ HR _____ P _____
Interval 5: TIME _____ HR _____ P _____

Workout Notes _____

Personal Notes _____

Wednesday ■ Date: ___ / ___ / ___

Waking Heart Rate _____

Standing Heart Rate _____

Waking Weight _____ Hours of Sleep _____

Quality of Sleep 1 2 3 4 5 6 7 8 9 10

Mood State 1 2 3 4 5 6 7 8 9 10

Goal _____

Workout _____

Specific Task _____

Actual Workout Time _____

Distance _____ Cadence _____

Average Heart Rate _____ Power _____

Interval 1: TIME _____ HR _____ P _____
Interval 2: TIME _____ HR _____ P _____
Interval 3: TIME _____ HR _____ P _____
Interval 4: TIME _____ HR _____ P _____
Interval 5: TIME _____ HR _____ P _____

Workout Notes _____

Personal Notes _____

Thursday ■ Date: ___ / ___ / ___

Waking Heart Rate ___

Standing Heart Rate ___

Waking Weight ___ Hours of Sleep ___

Quality of Sleep   1 2 3 4 5 6 7 8 9 10

Mood State   1 2 3 4 5 6 7 8 9 10

Goal ___

Workout ___

Specific Task ___

Actual Workout Time ___

Distance ___ Cadence ___

Average Heart Rate ___ Power ___

Interval 1: TIME ___ HR ___ P ___
Interval 2: TIME ___ HR ___ P ___
Interval 3: TIME ___ HR ___ P ___
Interval 4: TIME ___ HR ___ P ___
Interval 5: TIME ___ HR ___ P ___

Workout Notes ___

Personal Notes ___

Friday ■ Date: ___ / ___ / ___

Waking Heart Rate ___

Standing Heart Rate ___

Waking Weight ___ Hours of Sleep ___

Quality of Sleep   1 2 3 4 5 6 7 8 9 10

Mood State   1 2 3 4 5 6 7 8 9 10

Goal ___

Workout ___

Specific Task ___

Actual Workout Time ___

Distance ___ Cadence ___

Average Heart Rate ___ Power ___

Interval 1: TIME ___ HR ___ P ___
Interval 2: TIME ___ HR ___ P ___
Interval 3: TIME ___ HR ___ P ___
Interval 4: TIME ___ HR ___ P ___
Interval 5: TIME ___ HR ___ P ___

Workout Notes ___

Personal Notes ___

Saturday ■ Date: ___ / ___ / ___

Waking Heart Rate ___

Standing Heart Rate ___

Waking Weight ___ Hours of Sleep ___

Quality of Sleep   1 2 3 4 5 6 7 8 9 10

Mood State   1 2 3 4 5 6 7 8 9 10

Goal ___

Workout ___

Specific Task ___

Actual Workout Time ___

Distance ___ Cadence ___

Average Heart Rate ___ Power ___

Interval 1: TIME ___ HR ___ P ___
Interval 2: TIME ___ HR ___ P ___
Interval 3: TIME ___ HR ___ P ___
Interval 4: TIME ___ HR ___ P ___
Interval 5: TIME ___ HR ___ P ___

Workout Notes ___

Personal Notes ___

Sunday ■ Date: ___ / ___ / ___

Waking Heart Rate _____

Standing Heart Rate _____

Waking Weight _____ Hours of Sleep _____

Quality of Sleep 1 2 3 4 5 6 7 8 9 10

Mood State 1 2 3 4 5 6 7 8 9 10

Goal _____

Workout _____

Specific Task _____

Actual Workout Time _____

Distance _____ Cadence _____

Average Heart Rate _____ Power _____

Interval 1: TIME _____ HR _____ P _____

Interval 2: TIME _____ HR _____ P _____

Interval 3: TIME _____ HR _____ P _____

Interval 4: TIME _____ HR _____ P _____

Interval 5: TIME _____ HR _____ P _____

Workout Notes _____

Personal Notes _____

Weekly Summary

Hours of Cycling: _____ Year-to-Date: _____

Miles/Kilometers: _____ Year-to-Date: _____

Hours of Strength Training: _____ Year-to-Date: _____

Hours of Other Activities: _____ Year-to-Date: _____

_____ Year-to-Date: _____

_____ Year-to-Date: _____

_____ Year-to-Date: _____

Total Training Hours: _____

Number of Workouts Planned: _____

Number of Workouts Completed: _____

Average Hours of Sleep: _____

Average Quality of Sleep: _____

Average Mood State: _____

Time Spent in Heart Rate/Power Ranges:

CTS RANGES	TIME	CTS RANGES	TIME	OTHER WORKOUTS	TIME
RecoveryMiles™		SteadyState™			
FoundationMiles™		ClimbingRepeats™			
EnduranceMiles™		Max Effort			
Tempo™					

Personal Notes: _____

Weekly Strength Training Record

Exercise	Date:						Date:						Date:					
	SET 1		SET 2		SET 3		SET 1		SET 2		SET 3		SET 1		SET 2		SET 3	
	lbs.	reps	lbs.	reps	lbs.	reps	lbs.	reps	lbs.	reps	lbs.	reps	lbs.	reps	lbs.	reps	lbs.	reps

Race Results

Race #1 _____ Date: ___ / ___ / ___

Time _____ Distance _____

Goal _____

Result _____

Average Heart Rate _____ Power _____

Food/Fluid Intake _____

Personal Notes _____

Race #2 _____ Date: ___ / ___ / ___

Time _____ Distance _____

Goal _____

Result _____

Average Heart Rate _____ Power _____

Food/Fluid Intake _____

Personal Notes _____

Week #　　　　Goal:

Monday ▪ Date: ___ /___ /___

Waking Heart Rate

Standing Heart Rate

Waking Weight　　　　Hours of Sleep

Quality of Sleep　1 2 3 4 5 6 7 8 9 10

Mood State　1 2 3 4 5 6 7 8 9 10

Goal

Workout

Specific Task

Actual Workout Time

Distance　　　Cadence　　　

Average Heart Rate	Power
Interval 1:	TIME	HR ___ P ___
Interval 2:	TIME	HR ___ P ___
Interval 3:	TIME	HR ___ P ___
Interval 4:	TIME	HR ___ P ___
Interval 5:	TIME	HR ___ P ___

Workout Notes

Personal Notes

Tuesday ▪ Date: ___ /___ /___

Waking Heart Rate

Standing Heart Rate

Waking Weight　　　　Hours of Sleep

Quality of Sleep　1 2 3 4 5 6 7 8 9 10

Mood State　1 2 3 4 5 6 7 8 9 10

Goal

Workout

Specific Task

Actual Workout Time

Distance　　　Cadence　　　

Average Heart Rate	Power
Interval 1:	TIME	HR ___ P ___
Interval 2:	TIME	HR ___ P ___
Interval 3:	TIME	HR ___ P ___
Interval 4:	TIME	HR ___ P ___
Interval 5:	TIME	HR ___ P ___

Workout Notes

Personal Notes

Wednesday ▪ Date: ___ /___ /___

Waking Heart Rate

Standing Heart Rate

Waking Weight　　　　Hours of Sleep

Quality of Sleep　1 2 3 4 5 6 7 8 9 10

Mood State　1 2 3 4 5 6 7 8 9 10

Goal

Workout

Specific Task

Actual Workout Time

Distance　　　Cadence　　　

Average Heart Rate	Power
Interval 1:	TIME	HR ___ P ___
Interval 2:	TIME	HR ___ P ___
Interval 3:	TIME	HR ___ P ___
Interval 4:	TIME	HR ___ P ___
Interval 5:	TIME	HR ___ P ___

Workout Notes

Personal Notes

Week #

Thursday ▪ Date: ____ / ____ / ____

Waking Heart Rate _____

Standing Heart Rate _____

Waking Weight _____ Hours of Sleep _____

Quality of Sleep 1 2 3 4 5 6 7 8 9 10

Mood State 1 2 3 4 5 6 7 8 9 10

Goal _____

Workout _____

Specific Task _____

Actual Workout Time _____

Distance _____ Cadence _____

Average Heart Rate _____ Power _____

Interval 1: TIME _____ HR _____ P _____

Interval 2: TIME _____ HR _____ P _____

Interval 3: TIME _____ HR _____ P _____

Interval 4: TIME _____ HR _____ P _____

Interval 5: TIME _____ HR _____ P _____

Workout Notes _____

Personal Notes _____

Friday ▪ Date: ____ / ____ / ____

Waking Heart Rate _____

Standing Heart Rate _____

Waking Weight _____ Hours of Sleep _____

Quality of Sleep 1 2 3 4 5 6 7 8 9 10

Mood State 1 2 3 4 5 6 7 8 9 10

Goal _____

Workout _____

Specific Task _____

Actual Workout Time _____

Distance _____ Cadence _____

Average Heart Rate _____ Power _____

Interval 1: TIME _____ HR _____ P _____

Interval 2: TIME _____ HR _____ P _____

Interval 3: TIME _____ HR _____ P _____

Interval 4: TIME _____ HR _____ P _____

Interval 5: TIME _____ HR _____ P _____

Workout Notes _____

Personal Notes _____

Saturday ▪ Date: ____ / ____ / ____

Waking Heart Rate _____

Standing Heart Rate _____

Waking Weight _____ Hours of Sleep _____

Quality of Sleep 1 2 3 4 5 6 7 8 9 10

Mood State 1 2 3 4 5 6 7 8 9 10

Goal _____

Workout _____

Specific Task _____

Actual Workout Time _____

Distance _____ Cadence _____

Average Heart Rate _____ Power _____

Interval 1: TIME _____ HR _____ P _____

Interval 2: TIME _____ HR _____ P _____

Interval 3: TIME _____ HR _____ P _____

Interval 4: TIME _____ HR _____ P _____

Interval 5: TIME _____ HR _____ P _____

Workout Notes _____

Personal Notes _____

Week #

Sunday ■ Date: ___/___/___

Waking Heart Rate ___

Standing Heart Rate ___

Waking Weight ___ Hours of Sleep ___

Quality of Sleep   1 2 3 4 5 6 7 8 9 10

Mood State   1 2 3 4 5 6 7 8 9 10

Goal ___

Workout ___

Specific Task ___

Actual Workout Time ___

Distance ___ Cadence ___

Average Heart Rate ___ Power ___

Interval 1: TIME ___ HR ___ P ___
Interval 2: TIME ___ HR ___ P ___
Interval 3: TIME ___ HR ___ P ___
Interval 4: TIME ___ HR ___ P ___
Interval 5: TIME ___ HR ___ P ___

Workout Notes ___

Personal Notes ___

Weekly Summary

Hours of Cycling: ___ Year-to-Date: ___

Miles/Kilometers: ___ Year-to-Date: ___

Hours of Strength Training: ___ Year-to-Date: ___

Hours of Other Activities: ___

___ Year-to-Date: ___
___ Year-to-Date: ___
___ Year-to-Date: ___
___ Year-to-Date: ___

Total Training Hours: ___

Number of Workouts Planned: ___

Number of Workouts Completed: ___

Average Hours of Sleep: ___

Average Quality of Sleep: ___

Average Mood State: ___

Time Spent in Heart Rate/Power Ranges:

CTS RANGES	TIME	CTS RANGES	TIME	OTHER WORKOUTS	TIME
RecoveryMiles™		SteadyState™			
FoundationMiles™		ClimbingRepeats™			
EnduranceMiles™		Max Effort			
Tempo™					

Personal Notes: ___

| Week # | | Weekly Strength Training Record | | | | | | | | | | |

	Date:						Date:					Date:		
	SET 1		SET 2		SET 3		SET 1		SET 2		SET 3		SET 1		SET 2		SET 3
Exercise	lbs.	reps	lbs.	reps	lbs.	reps	lbs.	reps	lbs.	reps	lbs.	reps	lbs.	reps	lbs.	reps	lbs.	reps

Race Results

Race #1 _____ Date: ___/___/___

Time _____ Distance _____

Goal _____

Result _____

Average Heart Rate _____ Power _____

Food/Fluid Intake _____

Personal Notes _____

_____

_____

Race #2 _____ Date: ___/___/___

Time _____ Distance _____

Goal _____

Result _____

Average Heart Rate _____ Power _____

Food/Fluid Intake _____

Personal Notes _____

_____

_____

Week # _____   Goal: _____

Monday ▪ Date: ___/___/___

Waking Heart Rate _____
Standing Heart Rate _____
Waking Weight _____ Hours of Sleep _____
Quality of Sleep   1 2 3 4 5 6 7 8 9 10

Mood State   1 2 3 4 5 6 7 8 9 10

Goal _____
Workout _____
Specific Task _____
Actual Workout Time _____
Distance _____ Cadence _____

Average Heart Rate _____ Power _____
Interval 1: TIME _____ HR _____ P _____
Interval 2: TIME _____ HR _____ P _____
Interval 3: TIME _____ HR _____ P _____
Interval 4: TIME _____ HR _____ P _____
Interval 5: TIME _____ HR _____ P _____
Workout Notes _____

Personal Notes _____

Tuesday ▪ Date: ___/___/___

Waking Heart Rate _____
Standing Heart Rate _____
Waking Weight _____ Hours of Sleep _____
Quality of Sleep   1 2 3 4 5 6 7 8 9 10

Mood State   1 2 3 4 5 6 7 8 9 10

Goal _____
Workout _____
Specific Task _____
Actual Workout Time _____
Distance _____ Cadence _____

Average Heart Rate _____ Power _____
Interval 1: TIME _____ HR _____ P _____
Interval 2: TIME _____ HR _____ P _____
Interval 3: TIME _____ HR _____ P _____
Interval 4: TIME _____ HR _____ P _____
Interval 5: TIME _____ HR _____ P _____
Workout Notes _____

Personal Notes _____

Wednesday ▪ Date: ___/___/___

Waking Heart Rate _____
Standing Heart Rate _____
Waking Weight _____ Hours of Sleep _____
Quality of Sleep   1 2 3 4 5 6 7 8 9 10

Mood State   1 2 3 4 5 6 7 8 9 10

Goal _____
Workout _____
Specific Task _____
Actual Workout Time _____
Distance _____ Cadence _____

Average Heart Rate _____ Power _____
Interval 1: TIME _____ HR _____ P _____
Interval 2: TIME _____ HR _____ P _____
Interval 3: TIME _____ HR _____ P _____
Interval 4: TIME _____ HR _____ P _____
Interval 5: TIME _____ HR _____ P _____
Workout Notes _____

Personal Notes _____

Thursday ■ Date: ___ / ___ / ___

Waking Heart Rate _____

Standing Heart Rate _____

Waking Weight _____ Hours of Sleep _____

Quality of Sleep 1 2 3 4 5 6 7 8 9 10

Mood State 1 2 3 4 5 6 7 8 9 10

Goal _____

Workout _____

Specific Task _____

Actual Workout Time _____

Distance _____ Cadence _____

Average Heart Rate _____ Power _____

Interval 1: TIME _____ HR _____ P _____

Interval 2: TIME _____ HR _____ P _____

Interval 3: TIME _____ HR _____ P _____

Interval 4: TIME _____ HR _____ P _____

Interval 5: TIME _____ HR _____ P _____

Workout Notes _____

Personal Notes _____

Friday ■ Date: ___ / ___ / ___

Waking Heart Rate _____

Standing Heart Rate _____

Waking Weight _____ Hours of Sleep _____

Quality of Sleep 1 2 3 4 5 6 7 8 9 10

Mood State 1 2 3 4 5 6 7 8 9 10

Goal _____

Workout _____

Specific Task _____

Actual Workout Time _____

Distance _____ Cadence _____

Average Heart Rate _____ Power _____

Interval 1: TIME _____ HR _____ P _____

Interval 2: TIME _____ HR _____ P _____

Interval 3: TIME _____ HR _____ P _____

Interval 4: TIME _____ HR _____ P _____

Interval 5: TIME _____ HR _____ P _____

Workout Notes _____

Personal Notes _____

Saturday ■ Date: ___ / ___ / ___

Waking Heart Rate _____

Standing Heart Rate _____

Waking Weight _____ Hours of Sleep _____

Quality of Sleep 1 2 3 4 5 6 7 8 9 10

Mood State 1 2 3 4 5 6 7 8 9 10

Goal _____

Workout _____

Specific Task _____

Actual Workout Time _____

Distance _____ Cadence _____

Average Heart Rate _____ Power _____

Interval 1: TIME _____ HR _____ P _____

Interval 2: TIME _____ HR _____ P _____

Interval 3: TIME _____ HR _____ P _____

Interval 4: TIME _____ HR _____ P _____

Interval 5: TIME _____ HR _____ P _____

Workout Notes _____

Personal Notes _____

Week # _____

Sunday ▪ Date: ___ / ___ / ___

Waking Heart Rate _____

Standing Heart Rate _____

Waking Weight _____ Hours of Sleep _____

Quality of Sleep 1 2 3 4 5 6 7 8 9 10

Mood State 1 2 3 4 5 6 7 8 9 10

Goal _____

Workout _____

Specific Task _____

Actual Workout Time _____

Distance _____ Cadence _____

Average Heart Rate _____ Power _____

Interval 1:	TIME _____	HR _____	P _____
Interval 2:	TIME _____	HR _____	P _____
Interval 3:	TIME _____	HR _____	P _____
Interval 4:	TIME _____	HR _____	P _____
Interval 5:	TIME _____	HR _____	P _____

Workout Notes _____

Personal Notes _____

Weekly Summary

Hours of Cycling: _____ Year-to-Date: _____

Miles/Kilometers: _____ Year-to-Date: _____

Hours of Strength Training: _____ Year-to-Date: _____

Hours of Other Activities: _____

_____ Year-to-Date: _____

_____ Year-to-Date: _____

_____ Year-to-Date: _____

Total Training Hours: _____

Number of Workouts Planned: _____

Number of Workouts Completed: _____

Average Hours of Sleep: _____

Average Quality of Sleep: _____

Average Mood State: _____

Time Spent in Heart Rate/Power Ranges:

CTS RANGES	TIME	CTS RANGES	TIME	OTHER WORKOUTS	TIME
RecoveryMiles™	_____	SteadyState™	_____		_____
FoundationMiles™	_____	ClimbingRepeats™	_____		_____
EnduranceMiles™	_____	Max Effort	_____		_____
Tempo™	_____				

Personal Notes: _____

Weekly Strength Training Record

Exercise	Date:						Date:						Date:					
	SET 1		SET 2		SET 3		SET 1		SET 2		SET 3		SET 1		SET 2		SET 3	
	lbs.	reps	lbs.	reps	lbs.	reps	lbs.	reps	lbs.	reps	lbs.	reps	lbs.	reps	lbs.	reps	lbs.	reps

Race Results

Race #1 _____ Date: ___ / ___ / ___

Time _____ Distance _____

Goal _____

Result _____

Average Heart Rate _____ Power _____

Food/Fluid Intake _____

Personal Notes _____

_____

_____

Race #2 _____ Date: ___ / ___ / ___

Time _____ Distance _____

Goal _____

Result _____

Average Heart Rate _____ Power _____

Food/Fluid Intake _____

Personal Notes _____

_____

_____

Week # _____ Goal: _____

Monday ■ Date: ___ / ___ / ___

Waking Heart Rate _____

Standing Heart Rate _____

Waking Weight _____ Hours of Sleep _____

Quality of Sleep 1 2 3 4 5 6 7 8 9 10

Mood State 1 2 3 4 5 6 7 8 9 10

Goal _____

Workout _____

Specific Task _____

Actual Workout Time _____

Distance _____ Cadence _____

Average Heart Rate _____ Power _____

Interval 1: TIME _____ HR _____ P _____

Interval 2: TIME _____ HR _____ P _____

Interval 3: TIME _____ HR _____ P _____

Interval 4: TIME _____ HR _____ P _____

Interval 5: TIME _____ HR _____ P _____

Workout Notes _____

Personal Notes _____

Tuesday ■ Date: ___ / ___ / ___

Waking Heart Rate _____

Standing Heart Rate _____

Waking Weight _____ Hours of Sleep _____

Quality of Sleep 1 2 3 4 5 6 7 8 9 10

Mood State 1 2 3 4 5 6 7 8 9 10

Goal _____

Workout _____

Specific Task _____

Actual Workout Time _____

Distance _____ Cadence _____

Average Heart Rate _____ Power _____

Interval 1: TIME _____ HR _____ P _____

Interval 2: TIME _____ HR _____ P _____

Interval 3: TIME _____ HR _____ P _____

Interval 4: TIME _____ HR _____ P _____

Interval 5: TIME _____ HR _____ P _____

Workout Notes _____

Personal Notes _____

Wednesday ■ Date: ___ / ___ / ___

Waking Heart Rate _____

Standing Heart Rate _____

Waking Weight _____ Hours of Sleep _____

Quality of Sleep 1 2 3 4 5 6 7 8 9 10

Mood State 1 2 3 4 5 6 7 8 9 10

Goal _____

Workout _____

Specific Task _____

Actual Workout Time _____

Distance _____ Cadence _____

Average Heart Rate _____ Power _____

Interval 1: TIME _____ HR _____ P _____

Interval 2: TIME _____ HR _____ P _____

Interval 3: TIME _____ HR _____ P _____

Interval 4: TIME _____ HR _____ P _____

Interval 5: TIME _____ HR _____ P _____

Workout Notes _____

Personal Notes _____

Thursday ■ Date: ___ / ___ / ___

Waking Heart Rate ___

Standing Heart Rate ___

Waking Weight ___ Hours of Sleep ___

Quality of Sleep 1 2 3 4 5 6 7 8 9 10

Mood State 1 2 3 4 5 6 7 8 9 10

Goal ___

Workout ___

Specific Task ___

Actual Workout Time ___

Distance ___ Cadence ___

Average Heart Rate ___ Power ___

Interval 1: TIME ___ HR ___ P ___
Interval 2: TIME ___ HR ___ P ___
Interval 3: TIME ___ HR ___ P ___
Interval 4: TIME ___ HR ___ P ___
Interval 5: TIME ___ HR ___ P ___

Workout Notes ___

Personal Notes ___

Friday ■ Date: ___ / ___ / ___

Waking Heart Rate ___

Standing Heart Rate ___

Waking Weight ___ Hours of Sleep ___

Quality of Sleep 1 2 3 4 5 6 7 8 9 10

Mood State 1 2 3 4 5 6 7 8 9 10

Goal ___

Workout ___

Specific Task ___

Actual Workout Time ___

Distance ___ Cadence ___

Average Heart Rate ___ Power ___

Interval 1: TIME ___ HR ___ P ___
Interval 2: TIME ___ HR ___ P ___
Interval 3: TIME ___ HR ___ P ___
Interval 4: TIME ___ HR ___ P ___
Interval 5: TIME ___ HR ___ P ___

Workout Notes ___

Personal Notes ___

Saturday ■ Date: ___ / ___ / ___

Waking Heart Rate ___

Standing Heart Rate ___

Waking Weight ___ Hours of Sleep ___

Quality of Sleep 1 2 3 4 5 6 7 8 9 10

Mood State 1 2 3 4 5 6 7 8 9 10

Goal ___

Workout ___

Specific Task ___

Actual Workout Time ___

Distance ___ Cadence ___

Average Heart Rate ___ Power ___

Interval 1: TIME ___ HR ___ P ___
Interval 2: TIME ___ HR ___ P ___
Interval 3: TIME ___ HR ___ P ___
Interval 4: TIME ___ HR ___ P ___
Interval 5: TIME ___ HR ___ P ___

Workout Notes ___

Personal Notes ___

| Week # |

Sunday ■ Date: ___ / ___ / ___

Waking Heart Rate ___

Standing Heart Rate ___

Waking Weight ___ Hours of Sleep ___

Quality of Sleep 1 2 3 4 5 6 7 8 9 10

Mood State 1 2 3 4 5 6 7 8 9 10

Goal ___

Workout ___

Specific Task ___

Actual Workout Time ___

Distance ___ Cadence ___

Average Heart Rate ___ Power ___

Interval 1: TIME ___ HR ___ P ___

Interval 2: TIME ___ HR ___ P ___

Interval 3: TIME ___ HR ___ P ___

Interval 4: TIME ___ HR ___ P ___

Interval 5: TIME ___ HR ___ P ___

Workout Notes ___

Personal Notes ___

Weekly Summary

Hours of Cycling: ___ Year-to-Date: ___

Miles/Kilometers: ___ Year-to-Date: ___

Hours of Strength Training: ___ Year-to-Date: ___

Hours of Other Activities: ___ Year-to-Date: ___

___ Year-to-Date: ___

___ Year-to-Date: ___

Total Training Hours: ___ Year-to-Date: ___

Number of Workouts Planned: ___

Number of Workouts Completed: ___

Average Hours of Sleep: ___

Average Quality of Sleep: ___

Average Mood State: ___

Time Spent in Heart Rate/Power Ranges:

CTS RANGES	TIME	CTS RANGES	TIME	OTHER WORKOUTS	TIME
RecoveryMiles™		SteadyState™			
FoundationMiles™		ClimbingRepeats™			
EnduranceMiles™		Max Effort			
Tempo™					

Personal Notes: ___

Weekly Strength Training Record

Exercise	Date:						Date:						Date:					
	SET 1 lbs. / reps		SET 2 lbs. / reps		SET 3 lbs. / reps		SET 1 lbs. / reps		SET 2 lbs. / reps		SET 3 lbs. / reps		SET 1 lbs. / reps		SET 2 lbs. / reps		SET 3 lbs. / reps	

Race Results

Race #1 _____ Date: __ / __ / __

Time _____ Distance _____

Goal _____

Result _____

Average Heart Rate _____ Power _____

Food/Fluid Intake _____

Personal Notes _____

_____

_____

Race #2 _____ Date: __ / __ / __

Time _____ Distance _____

Goal _____

Result _____

Average Heart Rate _____ Power _____

Food/Fluid Intake _____

Personal Notes _____

_____

_____

Week # _____ Goal: _____

Monday ■ Date: ___ / ___ / ___

Waking Heart Rate _____

Standing Heart Rate _____

Waking Weight _____ Hours of Sleep _____

Quality of Sleep 1 2 3 4 5 6 7 8 9 10

Mood State 1 2 3 4 5 6 7 8 9 10

Goal _____

Workout _____

Specific Task _____

Actual Workout Time _____

Distance _____ Cadence _____ Power _____

Average Heart Rate _____

Interval 1: TIME _____ HR _____ P _____
Interval 2: TIME _____ HR _____ P _____
Interval 3: TIME _____ HR _____ P _____
Interval 4: TIME _____ HR _____ P _____
Interval 5: TIME _____ HR _____ P _____

Workout Notes _____

Personal Notes _____

Tuesday ■ Date: ___ / ___ / ___

Waking Heart Rate _____

Standing Heart Rate _____

Waking Weight _____ Hours of Sleep _____

Quality of Sleep 1 2 3 4 5 6 7 8 9 10

Mood State 1 2 3 4 5 6 7 8 9 10

Goal _____

Workout _____

Specific Task _____

Actual Workout Time _____

Distance _____ Cadence _____ Power _____

Average Heart Rate _____

Interval 1: TIME _____ HR _____ P _____
Interval 2: TIME _____ HR _____ P _____
Interval 3: TIME _____ HR _____ P _____
Interval 4: TIME _____ HR _____ P _____
Interval 5: TIME _____ HR _____ P _____

Workout Notes _____

Personal Notes _____

Wednesday ■ Date: ___ / ___ / ___

Waking Heart Rate _____

Standing Heart Rate _____

Waking Weight _____ Hours of Sleep _____

Quality of Sleep 1 2 3 4 5 6 7 8 9 10

Mood State 1 2 3 4 5 6 7 8 9 10

Goal _____

Workout _____

Specific Task _____

Actual Workout Time _____

Distance _____ Cadence _____ Power _____

Average Heart Rate _____

Interval 1: TIME _____ HR _____ P _____
Interval 2: TIME _____ HR _____ P _____
Interval 3: TIME _____ HR _____ P _____
Interval 4: TIME _____ HR _____ P _____
Interval 5: TIME _____ HR _____ P _____

Workout Notes _____

Personal Notes _____

Week #

Thursday ■ Date: ___ / ___ / ___

Waking Heart Rate ___

Standing Heart Rate ___

Waking Weight ___ Hours of Sleep ___

Quality of Sleep 1 2 3 4 5 6 7 8 9 10

Mood State 1 2 3 4 5 6 7 8 9 10

Goal ___

Workout ___

Specific Task ___

Actual Workout Time ___

Distance ___ Cadence ___

Average Heart Rate ___ Power ___

Interval 1: TIME ___ HR ___ P ___
Interval 2: TIME ___ HR ___ P ___
Interval 3: TIME ___ HR ___ P ___
Interval 4: TIME ___ HR ___ P ___
Interval 5: TIME ___ HR ___ P ___

Workout Notes ___

Personal Notes ___

Friday ■ Date: ___ / ___ / ___

Waking Heart Rate ___

Standing Heart Rate ___

Waking Weight ___ Hours of Sleep ___

Quality of Sleep 1 2 3 4 5 6 7 8 9 10

Mood State 1 2 3 4 5 6 7 8 9 10

Goal ___

Workout ___

Specific Task ___

Actual Workout Time ___

Distance ___ Cadence ___

Average Heart Rate ___ Power ___

Interval 1: TIME ___ HR ___ P ___
Interval 2: TIME ___ HR ___ P ___
Interval 3: TIME ___ HR ___ P ___
Interval 4: TIME ___ HR ___ P ___
Interval 5: TIME ___ HR ___ P ___

Workout Notes ___

Personal Notes ___

Saturday ■ Date: ___ / ___ / ___

Waking Heart Rate ___

Standing Heart Rate ___

Waking Weight ___ Hours of Sleep ___

Quality of Sleep 1 2 3 4 5 6 7 8 9 10

Mood State 1 2 3 4 5 6 7 8 9 10

Goal ___

Workout ___

Specific Task ___

Actual Workout Time ___

Distance ___ Cadence ___

Average Heart Rate ___ Power ___

Interval 1: TIME ___ HR ___ P ___
Interval 2: TIME ___ HR ___ P ___
Interval 3: TIME ___ HR ___ P ___
Interval 4: TIME ___ HR ___ P ___
Interval 5: TIME ___ HR ___ P ___

Workout Notes ___

Personal Notes ___

Week # _____

Sunday ■ Date: ____ / ____ / ____

Waking Heart Rate _____

Standing Heart Rate _____

Waking Weight _____ Hours of Sleep _____

Quality of Sleep 1 2 3 4 5 6 7 8 9 10

Mood State 1 2 3 4 5 6 7 8 9 10

Goal _____

Workout _____

Specific Task _____

Actual Workout Time _____

Distance _____ Cadence _____

Average Heart Rate _____ Power _____

Interval 1: TIME _____ HR _____ P _____

Interval 2: TIME _____ HR _____ P _____

Interval 3: TIME _____ HR _____ P _____

Interval 4: TIME _____ HR _____ P _____

Interval 5: TIME _____ HR _____ P _____

Workout Notes _____

Personal Notes _____

Weekly Summary

Hours of Cycling: _____ Year-to-Date: _____

Miles/Kilometers: _____ Year-to-Date: _____

Hours of Strength Training: _____ Year-to-Date: _____

Hours of Other Activities: _____

_____ Year-to-Date: _____

_____ Year-to-Date: _____

_____ Year-to-Date: _____

_____ Year-to-Date: _____

Total Training Hours: _____

Number of Workouts Planned: _____

Number of Workouts Completed: _____

Average Hours of Sleep: _____

Average Quality of Sleep: _____

Average Mood State: _____

Time Spent in Heart Rate/Power Ranges:

CTS RANGES	TIME	CTS RANGES	TIME	OTHER WORKOUTS	TIME
RecoveryMiles™	_____	SteadyState™	_____	_____	_____
FoundationMiles™	_____	ClimbingRepeats™	_____	_____	_____
EnduranceMiles™	_____	Max Effort	_____	_____	_____
Tempo™	_____				

Personal Notes: _____

Weekly Strength Training Record

Exercise	Date:						Date:						Date:					
	SET 1		SET 2		SET 3		SET 1		SET 2		SET 3		SET 1		SET 2		SET 3	
	lbs.	reps	lbs.	reps	lbs.	reps	lbs.	reps	lbs.	reps	lbs.	reps	lbs.	reps	lbs.	reps	lbs.	reps

Race Results

Race #1 _____ Date: __/__/__

Time _____ Distance _____

Goal _____

Result _____

Average Heart Rate _____ Power _____

Food/Fluid Intake _____

Personal Notes _____

_____

_____

Race #2 _____ Date: __/__/__

Time _____ Distance _____

Goal _____

Result _____

Average Heart Rate _____ Power _____

Food/Fluid Intake _____

Personal Notes _____

_____

_____

Week # _____   Goal: _____

Monday ■ Date: ___ / ___ / ___

Waking Heart Rate _____

Standing Heart Rate _____

Waking Weight _____ Hours of Sleep _____

Quality of Sleep 1 2 3 4 5 6 7 8 9 10

Mood State 1 2 3 4 5 6 7 8 9 10

Goal _____

Workout _____

Specific Task _____

Actual Workout Time _____

Distance _____ Cadence _____

Average Heart Rate _____ Power _____

Interval 1: TIME _____ HR _____ P _____

Interval 2: TIME _____ HR _____ P _____

Interval 3: TIME _____ HR _____ P _____

Interval 4: TIME _____ HR _____ P _____

Interval 5: TIME _____ HR _____ P _____

Workout Notes _____

Personal Notes _____

Tuesday ■ Date: ___ / ___ / ___

Waking Heart Rate _____

Standing Heart Rate _____

Waking Weight _____ Hours of Sleep _____

Quality of Sleep 1 2 3 4 5 6 7 8 9 10

Mood State 1 2 3 4 5 6 7 8 9 10

Goal _____

Workout _____

Specific Task _____

Actual Workout Time _____

Distance _____ Cadence _____

Average Heart Rate _____ Power _____

Interval 1: TIME _____ HR _____ P _____

Interval 2: TIME _____ HR _____ P _____

Interval 3: TIME _____ HR _____ P _____

Interval 4: TIME _____ HR _____ P _____

Interval 5: TIME _____ HR _____ P _____

Workout Notes _____

Personal Notes _____

Wednesday ■ Date: ___ / ___ / ___

Waking Heart Rate _____

Standing Heart Rate _____

Waking Weight _____ Hours of Sleep _____

Quality of Sleep 1 2 3 4 5 6 7 8 9 10

Mood State 1 2 3 4 5 6 7 8 9 10

Goal _____

Workout _____

Specific Task _____

Actual Workout Time _____

Distance _____ Cadence _____

Average Heart Rate _____ Power _____

Interval 1: TIME _____ HR _____ P _____

Interval 2: TIME _____ HR _____ P _____

Interval 3: TIME _____ HR _____ P _____

Interval 4: TIME _____ HR _____ P _____

Interval 5: TIME _____ HR _____ P _____

Workout Notes _____

Personal Notes _____

Week #

Thursday ■ Date: ___ / ___ / ___

Waking Heart Rate _____

Standing Heart Rate _____

Waking Weight _____ Hours of Sleep _____

Quality of Sleep 1 2 3 4 5 6 7 8 9 10

Mood State 1 2 3 4 5 6 7 8 9 10

Goal _____

Workout _____

Specific Task _____

Actual Workout Time _____

Distance _____ Cadence _____

Average Heart Rate _____ Power _____

Interval 1: TIME _____ HR _____ P _____
Interval 2: TIME _____ HR _____ P _____
Interval 3: TIME _____ HR _____ P _____
Interval 4: TIME _____ HR _____ P _____
Interval 5: TIME _____ HR _____ P _____

Workout Notes _____

Personal Notes _____

Friday ■ Date: ___ / ___ / ___

Waking Heart Rate _____

Standing Heart Rate _____

Waking Weight _____ Hours of Sleep _____

Quality of Sleep 1 2 3 4 5 6 7 8 9 10

Mood State 1 2 3 4 5 6 7 8 9 10

Goal _____

Workout _____

Specific Task _____

Actual Workout Time _____

Distance _____ Cadence _____

Average Heart Rate _____ Power _____

Interval 1: TIME _____ HR _____ P _____
Interval 2: TIME _____ HR _____ P _____
Interval 3: TIME _____ HR _____ P _____
Interval 4: TIME _____ HR _____ P _____
Interval 5: TIME _____ HR _____ P _____

Workout Notes _____

Personal Notes _____

Saturday ■ Date: ___ / ___ / ___

Waking Heart Rate _____

Standing Heart Rate _____

Waking Weight _____ Hours of Sleep _____

Quality of Sleep 1 2 3 4 5 6 7 8 9 10

Mood State 1 2 3 4 5 6 7 8 9 10

Goal _____

Workout _____

Specific Task _____

Actual Workout Time _____

Distance _____ Cadence _____

Average Heart Rate _____ Power _____

Interval 1: TIME _____ HR _____ P _____
Interval 2: TIME _____ HR _____ P _____
Interval 3: TIME _____ HR _____ P _____
Interval 4: TIME _____ HR _____ P _____
Interval 5: TIME _____ HR _____ P _____

Workout Notes _____

Personal Notes _____

Week # _____

Sunday ■ Date: _____ / _____ / _____

Waking Heart Rate _____

Standing Heart Rate _____

Waking Weight _____ Hours of Sleep _____

Quality of Sleep   1 2 3 4 5 6 7 8 9 10

Mood State   1 2 3 4 5 6 7 8 9 10

Goal _____

Workout _____

Specific Task _____

Actual Workout Time _____

Distance _____ Cadence _____

Average Heart Rate _____ Power _____

Interval 1: TIME _____ HR _____ P _____

Interval 2: TIME _____ HR _____ P _____

Interval 3: TIME _____ HR _____ P _____

Interval 4: TIME _____ HR _____ P _____

Interval 5: TIME _____ HR _____ P _____

Workout Notes _____

Personal Notes _____

Weekly Summary

Hours of Cycling: _____ Year-to-Date: _____

Miles/Kilometers: _____ Year-to-Date: _____

Hours of Strength Training: _____ Year-to-Date: _____

Hours of Other Activities: _____ Year-to-Date: _____

_____ Year-to-Date: _____

_____ Year-to-Date: _____

_____ Year-to-Date: _____

_____ Year-to-Date: _____

Total Training Hours: _____

Number of Workouts Planned: _____

Number of Workouts Completed: _____

Average Hours of Sleep: _____

Average Quality of Sleep: _____

Average Mood State: _____

Time Spent in Heart Rate/Power Ranges:

CTS RANGES	TIME	CTS RANGES	TIME	OTHER WORKOUTS	TIME
RecoveryMiles™	_____	SteadyState™	_____	_____	_____
FoundationMiles™	_____	ClimbingRepeats™	_____	_____	_____
EnduranceMiles™	_____	Max Effort	_____	_____	_____
Tempo™	_____				

Personal Notes: _____

Weekly Strength Training Record

Exercise	Date:						Date:						Date:					
	SET 1		SET 2		SET 3		SET 1		SET 2		SET 3		SET 1		SET 2		SET 3	
	lbs.	reps	lbs.	reps	lbs.	reps	lbs.	reps	lbs.	reps	lbs.	reps	lbs.	reps	lbs.	reps	lbs.	reps

Race Results

Race #1 _____ Date: ___ / ___ / ___

Time _____ Distance _____

Goal _____

Result _____

Average Heart Rate _____ Power _____

Food/Fluid Intake _____

Personal Notes _____
_____
_____
_____

Race #2 _____ Date: ___ / ___ / ___

Time _____ Distance _____

Goal _____

Result _____

Average Heart Rate _____ Power _____

Food/Fluid Intake _____

Personal Notes _____
_____
_____
_____

Part 3:

Appendix

CTS Field Tests

When performing a CTS Field Test, collect the following data:

- Time of each effort (mm:ss)
- Average heart rate for each effort
- Average power (if available) for each effort
- Average cadence for each effort
- Weather conditions (warm vs. cold, windy vs. calm, etc.)
- Course conditions (indoors vs. outdoors, flat vs. hilly, point-to-point vs. out and back, etc.)
- Rate of Perceived Exertion (RPE) (how hard you felt you were working) for each effort.

You are going to repeat this field test several times throughout the year, and the data you gather need to be comparable between tests. Repeated field tests establish baseline data you can use to evaluate your training progress. The more consistent you keep your field test location and conditions, the more accurately you can judge your progress over time. Try to reduce the number of variables between tests by using the same course under similar conditions (temperature, wind) every time.

Step One: Find a test course. Locate and measure a flat three-mile course or a two- to three-mile climb.

Step Two: Warm up and start the ride right. Ride hard enough to sweat for 10 to 20 minutes, but don't go as hard as you can. Select a gear that allows a quick, stable start. Don't start too fast—give yourself at least one minute to reach top speed.

Step Three: Find your ideal gear and feel the burn. Select a gear that allows you to maintain a cadence between 90–95 RPM (crank revolutions per minute) on flat terrain and 80–85 RPMs when climbing. Avoid the impulse to mash a big gear at low RPM. Settle into a steady rhythm of breathing. From here it's going to hurt. If it isn't challenging at this point, you need to pedal harder and faster.

Step Four: Recover and repeat. Once you're done the first effort, take 10–15 minutes recovery time before you repeat it. Complete your second field test effort and record your data. You're done! Ride easy for 15–30 minutes and then go home.

Use the following table to record your results from CTS Field Tests:

CTS Field Tests

Date	Test	Elapsed Time	Avg HR	Max HR	Avg Power	Max Power	Avg Cadence	RPE	Weather Conditions/Course Conditions/Notes
8/15/04	Effort 1	8:02	185	197	250	425	90	9	Sunny, 75
	Effort 2	8:12	185	197	250	425	90	9	Out and back
	Effort 1								
	Effort 2								
	Effort 1								
	Effort 2								
	Effort 1								
	Effort 2								
	Effort 1								
	Effort 2								
	Effort 1								
	Effort 2								
	Effort 1								
	Effort 2								

Date	Test	Elapsed Time	Avg HR	Max HR	Avg Power	Max Power	Avg Cadence	RPE	Weather Conditions/Course Conditions/Notes	
8/15/04	Effort 1	8:02	185	197	250	425	90	9	Sunny, 75	
	Effort 2	8:12	185	197	250	425	90	9	Out and back	
	Effort 1									
	Effort 2									
	Effort 1									
	Effort 2									
	Effort 1									
	Effort 2									
	Effort 1									
	Effort 2									
	Effort 1									
	Effort 2									
	Effort 1									
	Effort 2									

Test Results

Date	Test	Results

Event Results

Date	Event Name	Event Type (road, mtn., etc.)	Distance	Placement	Points Earned

Do-It-Yourself Graphs

Use these grids to plot whatever you want. You can use it to see how your waking weight changed over the course of February, or you may decide to use it to build a graphic representation of your training hours for the month.

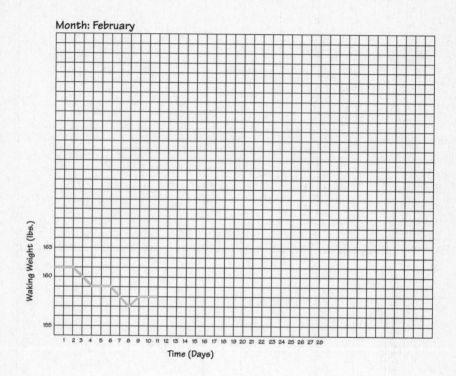

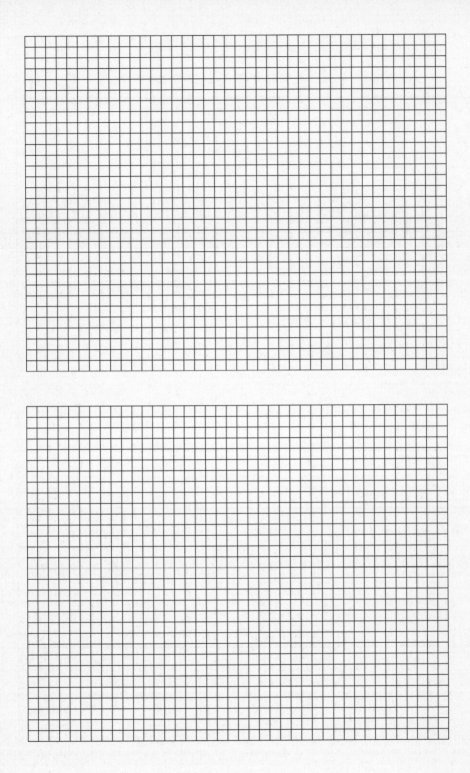

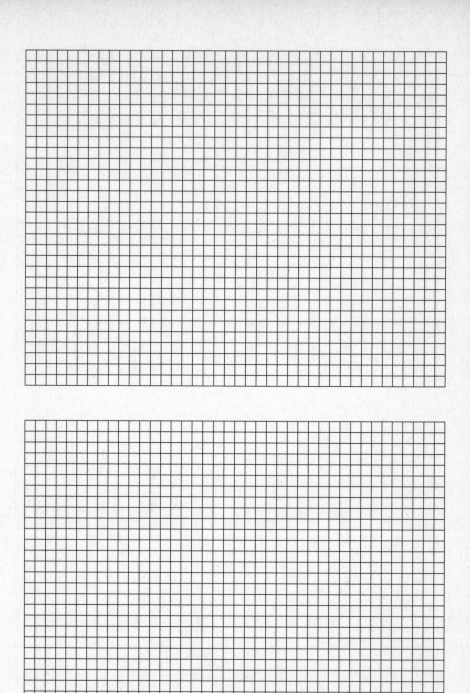

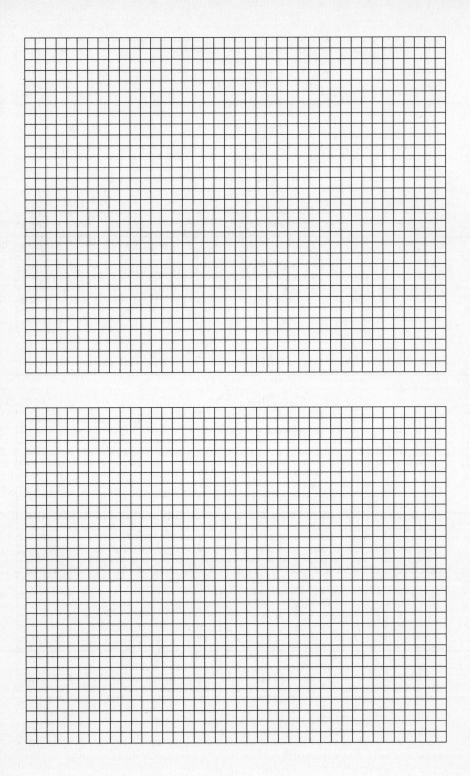

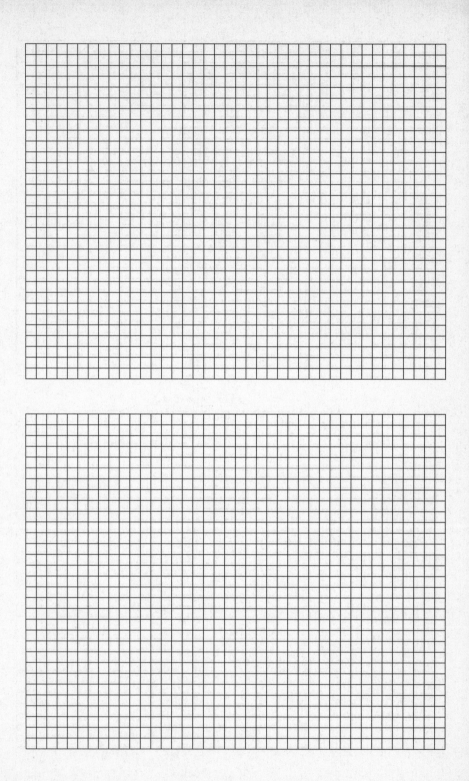

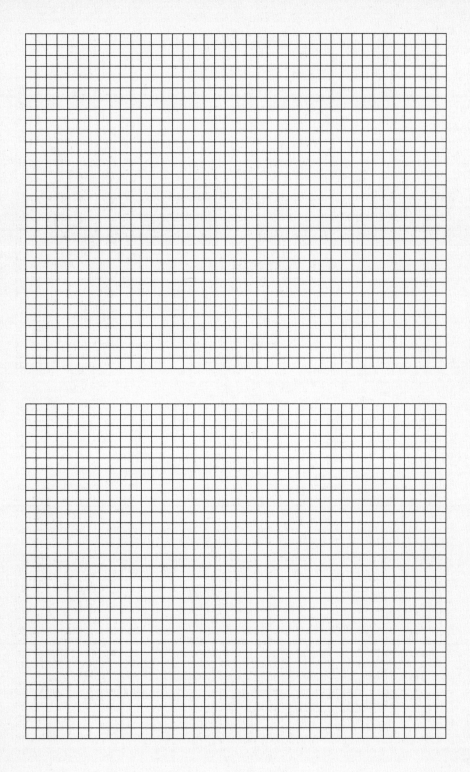

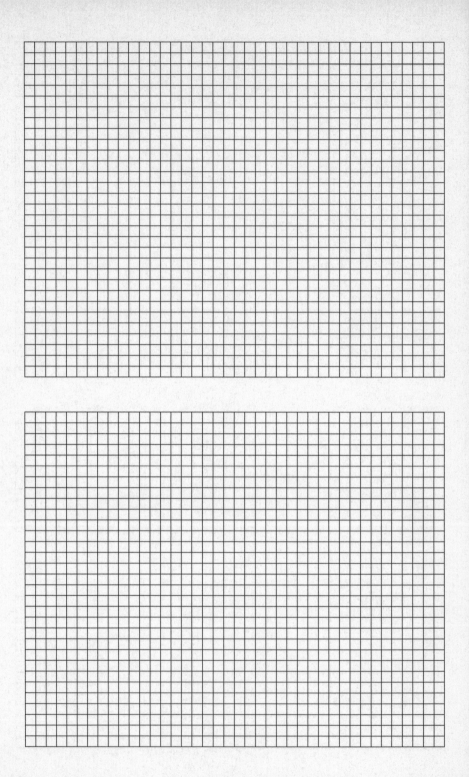

Bike Fit

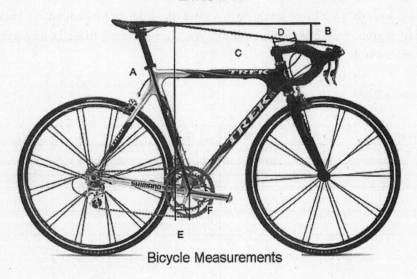

Bicycle Measurements

A = Seat height (middle of bottom bracket to top of saddle, along the line of the seat tube)

B = Vertical difference between top of saddle and top of bars

C = Ultimate reach: Tip of saddle to tip of brakehood

D = Length of stem

E = Seat setback (horizontal distance from tip of saddle and center of bottom bracket)

F = Crank length (center of bottom bracket to the center of the pedal spindle)

Bike/Date	A	B	C	D	E	F

Many cyclists ride more than one bicycle, and it's important to keep track of the bike fit measurements for your mountain bike, second road bike, triathlon bike, and/or track bike. If you have a time trial bike, or you adjust the fit of your regular road bike for time trials, you should record these fit measurements as well.

Bicycle 2: _____

Bike/Date	A	B	C	D	E	F

Bicycle 3: _____

Bike/Date	A	B	C	D	E	F

Equipment Log

Equipment	Date Installed	Cost	Purchased	Replaced	Repaired

Pre-Event Checklist

Equipment
- ❑ bike (race ready)
- ❑ helmet
- ❑ heart rate monitor
- ❑ trainer/rollers
- ❑ floor pump
- ❑ pit wheels
- ❑ training tires
- ❑ spare tires
- ❑ spare tubes
- ❑ extra cleats
- ❑ tool kit
- ❑ lubricant
- ❑ extra cassette

Clothing
- ❑ short-sleeve race jersey
- ❑ long-sleeve race jersey
- ❑ race shorts or race bibs
- ❑ skinsuit
- ❑ base layer
- ❑ sports bra
- ❑ socks
- ❑ arm warmers
- ❑ knee warmers
- ❑ leg warmers
- ❑ tights
- ❑ vest
- ❑ windbreaker
- ❑ rain jacket
- ❑ fingerless gloves
- ❑ windproof gloves
- ❑ sunglasses
- ❑ spare lenses
- ❑ cycling shoes
- ❑ shoe covers
- ❑ casual clothes

Food/Liquids
- ❑ water bottles
- ❑ water (1–2 gallons)
- ❑ CTS/PowerBar
- ❑ Endurance and Recovery drink mixes
- ❑ PowerBars
- ❑ PowerGel
- ❑ solid food

Miscellaneous
- ❑ racing license
- ❑ safety pins
- ❑ directions to the race

- ❑ first-aid kit
- ❑ warm-up liniments
- ❑ chamois cream
- ❑ towel
- ❑ extra money

Other
- ❑ _____
- ❑ _____
- ❑ _____
- ❑ _____
- ❑ _____
- ❑ _____
- ❑ _____
- ❑ _____
- ❑ _____
- ❑ _____
- ❑ _____
- ❑ _____
- ❑ _____
- ❑ _____
- ❑ _____
- ❑ _____
- ❑ _____
- ❑ _____
- ❑ _____
- ❑ _____

Contact Information

Coach _____

Phone (w)_____

Phone (c) _____

Email _____

Website _____

Local Bike Shop_____

Phone (w)_____

Phone (c) _____

Email _____

Website _____

Local Cycling Association

_____

Phone_____

Email _____

Website _____

Representative _____

Phone_____

Email _____

Membership #_____

Team_____

Website _____

Name _____

Phone (w)_____

Phone (c) _____

Phone (h) _____

Email _____

Name _____

Phone (w)_____

Phone (c) _____

Phone (h) _____

Email _____

Name _____

Phone (w)_____

Phone (c) _____

Phone (h) _____

Email _____

Name _____

Phone (w)_____

Phone (c) _____

Phone (h) _____

Email _____

Name _____

Phone (w)_____

Phone (c) _____

Phone (h) _____

Email _____

Other Contacts

Name _____

Phone_____

Email _____

Website _____

Name _____

Phone_____

Email _____

Website _____

Name _____

Phone_____

Email _____

Website _____

Carmichael Training Systems

719.635.0645

www.trainright.com

Notes:

_____

_____

_____

_____

_____

_____

_____